Praise for *Cheating Death*

"Getting older is no longer about treating symptoms and conditions, it's about extending your mental and physical vitality and feeling better longer. Dr. Rand McClain is a worldwide expert when it comes to the newest therapies and technologies that can help extend healthspan and make aging something to enjoy."

—**Hal Elrod, author, speaker, and founder of The Miracle Morning Community**

"*Cheating Death* is a great title, but it's not what this book is about. This book is about LIVING LIFE, especially as we get older. As a 54-year-old Sleep Doctor, not only am I taking his advice about nutrition, movement, etc, but after careful review of his writings on sleep, I can tell you, this book has exactly what we all need, to live longer, happier, and healthier lives."

—**Dr. Michael Breus, PhD, D, ABSM (Diplomate, American Board of Sleep Medicine) and founder of TheSleepDoctor.com**

"Dr. Rand McClain is our go-to source for information regarding medical treatments for anti-aging, longevity, improving physical performance, and health. In a field that is rife with misinformation, especially around hormone therapy, Dr. Rand is a welcome breath of fresh air. When Dr. Rand talks, I listen."

—**Sal DiStefano, cofounder of Mind Pump Media and cohost of Mind Pump**

"Death is something we all will face. *Cheating Death* outlines options, protocols, and advancements in medicine—both traditional and alternative—that can help us push past some of the conditions that can lead to premature death."

—**Dr. Kami Hoss, DDS, MS, cofounder of The Super Dentists, Howard Healthcare Academy, and SuperMouth™, author of *If Your Mouth Could Talk***

"The information in this book gives us permission to think differently about our expectations around quality of life in the final decades and enhance function and performance no matter what our age."

—**Jill Carnahan, MD, ABIHM, ABoIM, IFMCP, functional medicine expert at Flatiron Functional Medicine**

"It never ceases to amaze me the amount of time and money people spend on things that will shorten their lives and ruin their quality of life. Unhealthy processed food, alcohol, cigarettes/vaping. But you mention stem cell therapy or hormone replacement therapy and they start backing away out of fear of the boogie man. *Cheating Death* explains the latest scientific breakthroughs in longevity. You deserve not just to live a life but to live your best possible life and that's exactly what Dr. Rand McClain's book is all about. Think of it as an investment in yourself."

—**Duffy Gaver, master trainer to the stars and author of *Hero Maker: 12 Weeks to Superhero Fit: A Hollywood Trainer's REAL Guide to Getting the Body You've Always Wanted***

"Dr. Rand McClain provides a very timely and comprehensive book on ways to live longer and live better. His unique perspective as a patient and a physician offers the reader a clear and easily understandable approach to preventing disease and optimizing wellness. This is a must-read for anyone wanting to learn the latest science and breakthroughs on health and wellness."

—Dr. Nathan S. Bryan, author, entrepreneur, and nitric oxide biochemist

CHEATING DEATH

THE NEW SCIENCE OF LIVING LONGER AND BETTER

RAND McCLAIN, DO

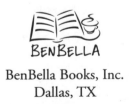

BenBella Books, Inc.
Dallas, TX

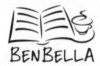

BenBella Books, Inc.
10440 N. Central Expressway
Suite 800
Dallas, TX 75231
benbellabooks.com
Send feedback to feedback@benbellabooks.com

BenBella is a federally registered trademark.

Printed in the United States of America
10 9 8 7 6 5 4 3 2 1

Library of Congress Control Number: 2022033391
ISBN 9781637740408 (hardcover)
eISBN 9781637740415

Editing by Brian Nicol
Copyediting by James Fraleigh
Proofreading by Kellie Doherty and Rebecca Maines
Indexing by WordCo
Text design and composition by PerfecType, Nashville, TN
Cover design by Lara Frayre
Cover image © Shutterstock / Vadarshop (DNA), STOP_WAR (DNA ring), Trikona (mandala), and Pavel Kubarkov (grainy texture); Unsplash / Kier in Sight (gold glitter); and YouWorkForThem / RuleByArt (chroma)
Printed by Lake Book Manufacturing

Special discounts for bulk sales are available. Please contact bulkorders@benbellabooks.com.

To those who consider not just probability, but also possibility.
And to those who never quit their estimable pursuits.

CONTENTS

PART III
FOUR ANTI-AGING TOOLS FOR LEVELING
THE LONGEVITY PLAYING FIELD

PART IV
LIVING LONGER AND BETTER WITH HORMONES

PART V
CHEATING DEATH WITH TECHNOLOGY, ANALYTICS, AND ACTION

INTRODUCTION

HEALTHSPAN REPRESENTS THE combination of health and lifespan. Years ago, the goal was to live longer. Now that many of us are living to age eighty and well beyond, we want more than quantity—we want quality. We hope to feel and look good as we get older, we aspire to heal from injuries and illness faster, and we expect to have the energy to do what we wish—from work to exercise to sex.

Traditional medicine provides various medications and procedures designed to enhance our healthspan, but these have little to offer. Sometimes, insurance companies refuse to reimburse approaches they deem "experimental." Sometimes, the US Food and Drug Administration (FDA) is slow to approve effective products and treatments, requiring years of rigorous studies and tests. Sometimes, there's no money in a given product or procedure—if Big Pharma doesn't anticipate a lot of profit, they ignore it and don't use their marketing muscle to spread the word. And, in certain instances, doctors and other healthcare practitioners are slow to accept new and emerging methods. Some physicians cling to what they've used for years and are reluctant to embrace a new or unconventional product or technique—sometimes for good reasons and sometimes for bad ones.

The good news is, despite these obstacles, healthspan-boosting approaches are proliferating, helping us live longer, heal faster, and feel better. I hope to use this book to spread the word about these approaches so that a growing number of people can take advantage of them. I call these approaches the means by which we are "cheating Death."

My motivation is both personal and professional. In terms of the latter, I am a medical doctor whose Regenerative & Sports Medicine Clinic in Santa Monica, California, is well known as a leading center of alternative (meaning science based, but not necessarily "mainstream") and cutting-edge treatments—from cryotherapy to bioidentical hormone replacement therapy to hyperbaric oxygen therapy. We have attracted a wide range of patients, not just from Southern California, but from around the world—entrepreneurs, celebrities, world-class athletes, and many others searching for effective and innovative treatments. I'll share these treatments with you, helping you understand the science behind them while showing you how to benefit from them in your own life.

Can we really cheat Death? Not indefinitely, of course, but this book's title is meant to be thought-provoking. New and emerging discoveries are making it possible to delay our inevitable decline. We can cheat Death in the sense that we can spot and even prevent diseases earlier that might have killed us only a few years ago, we can take supplements and medications that can restore everything from our libidos to our energy, and we can use diet or extreme temperatures to look and feel better than previous generations. Ultimately, the intention is to not only "cheat Death" by adding years to our lives, but also to ensure that they are healthful and happy years worth living, which is just as important.

The book is divided into five parts. The first part introduces you to the concept of healthspan and the theories about aging that underlie it as well as "products" like supplements, nutrition, and other things that can be swallowed, injected, or infused to create positive healthspan effects. The second part focuses on a range of therapies that emphasize mobility advantage, including an in-depth look at stem and Muse cell therapy, whole-body cold and heat therapy, and hyperbaric oxygen therapy. Part three examines four health tools that level the longevity playing field—metformin, peptides, rapamycin, and nitric oxide—while part four follows up with a discussion of hormone replacement therapies, specifically bioidentical hormone replacement therapy, or BHRT. Last, part five examines a variety of emerging methods and technologies that can improve how long and well we live, such as early detection and diagnosis, gene editing, and various wearables or mobile applications that are revolutionizing the way we track, store, and use health data.

Personally, I'm driven to write this book because the treatments I'll discuss have not only helped my patients heal and feel better, they have also saved *my* life. Though I typically keep my own story private—I prefer to focus on the science and the treatment advice—I want to communicate that I'm not just a doctor, but also a patient. I have experienced various injuries and illnesses and, by being up front about what I've gone through, I think I can communicate why I'm so passionate about this subject.

A BRIEF HISTORY OF THE DOCTOR AS PATIENT

Most of my life, I've been cheating Death.

My first surgery was at age five to remove my tonsils and adenoids. The anesthesia mask was placed on my face, but the anesthesiologist apparently forgot to turn on the oxygen and eventual gas flow, because I couldn't breathe. I kept wondering what I had done wrong that my parents had sent me to this room to be suffocated by a man who only pressed harder on my face with the mask the more I struggled to breathe. As you might imagine, I was terrified at even the thought of any surgical procedures after that experience. Death was coming for me, I was sure. Strike one for my confidence in surgical medicine.

My next surgery was an emergency. I was feeling under the weather while a student at Washington and Lee University, and I made a last-minute dash after lunch to the infirmary to see what might be making me feel sick and lose my typically voracious appetite. The doctor put me through the usual paces and, suspecting appendicitis as one of the possibilities, pressed on McBurney's point (which is used to help diagnose appendicitis) on the lower right quadrant of my abdomen and asked me to jump up and down.

My pain tolerance has always been extremely high—I was the kid who went about my business with a broken arm for a couple of weeks, not once, but twice, before my parents asked me why I was eating with my nondominant hand. So, when the doctor pressed and I jumped, I didn't react.

He then ordered a CBC STAT (a complete blood count that includes a white blood cell count that, if elevated, would indicate appendicitis; STAT means "right away" in med–speak). Meanwhile, he called my pediatrician, who relayed the broken-bone stories and explained that if I was complaining about anything, it was most likely significant. Sure enough, the lab assays suggested appendicitis and I was sent by ambulance to the local hospital for an emergency appendectomy. The anesthesiologist said that while she could offer me general anesthesia, I would be safer undergoing a spinal nerve block instead because I had just eaten lunch, increasing the risk of throwing up while unconscious and inhaling the vomit, which can cause death. *Easy choice*, I thought.

After my spinal injection, the anesthesiologist appeared anxious—I followed her gaze to the blood-spattered wall behind me. *No biggie*, I thought, *just like me to make a mess.* Several minutes later, the OR nurse who was trying to gauge whether the spinal anesthesia was working got aggravated with me when I answered that I felt her pin-prick the same on my arm as I did my abdomen.

"Are you sure you aren't just feeling the pressure of my pin on your abdomen rather than a sharp sensation," she asked.

"Nope, it's equally sharp," I said.

Finally, she asked if it felt "exactly the same on my arm as on my abdomen."

I answered, "Well, no, not *exactly* like each other." That answer seemed to satisfy her that the spinal injection was working, so she brought the surgeon over to the OR table to begin the appendectomy.

When I stated that I could tell that she was swabbing my abdomen with gauze rather than cotton swabs because I could feel the texture, I saw my surgeon's eyes open wide and look over my head at the anesthesiologist. Still, for reasons unknown to me, everyone was satisfied that the anesthesia was working and, a few minutes later, it was time to cut.

At this point, even with the high pain threshold I inherited from my mother, I felt the excruciating sharpness of the scalpel slicing into my belly and told the surgeon so. He ordered the anesthesiologist to add IV painkillers equivalent to Darvon and Percocet that "could sedate an elephant" (or so they later told me) and tilted the OR table downward (the "Trendelenburg position") toward my head.

Because of the pain, my abdominal muscles had reacted by becoming taut, preventing the surgeon from cutting deeper into my abdomen for the appendix. The surgeon therefore ordered general anesthesia. Recalling the danger of having this anesthesia after a meal, I resisted. Despite the IV medications, I was later told that it took five people to pin me down so that they could place the mask on my face to administer the gas. Death was coming for me again.

They removed my appendix, and the last thing that I remember before losing consciousness was the doctor saying, "About two minutes more and it likely would have burst." Then, while I was in the post-op area, one of two things happened: either my chart did not mention the spinal block or the post-op nurse saw that I had undergone anesthesia and assumed no block had been administered. Either way, in keeping with the standard of care back then, I was asked to stand up shortly after awakening and to cough several times while standing. The problem: standing and coughing can cause a leak in the spinal cord's covering and a loss of

CSF (cerebrospinal fluid)—hence, why it's no longer the standard of care. That's just what I experienced, and the leak produced weeks of severe headaches and malaise. Strike two.

A year or so later, I developed a severely herniated disc in my cervical (neck) spine, and when my doctor suggested surgery to repair it, I said that would happen only if I were close to my last breath. I was still in college and a member of one of our US National water polo teams with access to some of the best doctors in the world, and they all said the same thing. Back then, the only options were fusion (essentially bolting the vertebrae together where the injury is) or an early-stage "disc replacement," which was at best the equivalent of a door hinge. *No way.*

A number of years later, I tried to squat my way to 260 pounds overnight, but during one training session, while struggling to do another repetition, I began leaning forward and looked to the ceiling to straighten up my form. I don't remember a snap—or much of anything—but that's when I really further injured my neck.

I saw a number of doctors and the eleventh one at that point, neurologist Glen Morrison, told me what I wanted to hear: "Don't baby it, just get back in there and like getting water flowing through a water hose, the more water you get moving through it the more you will help unkink the hose."

Perfect! And, it seemed to work for the next thirty-three years, despite the warnings I received from the other doctors that from then on, I would only be able to walk or maybe swim for exercise and that I would be in a wheelchair by the time I reached forty. I returned to the gym about six months after my initial diagnosis and was squatting 365 pounds for twelve reps like I was going for a walk in the park. Though I did experience chronic pain and an odd, occasional electric jolt during this time, their predictions never came to pass.

Thirty-three years later I was training as an Olympic lifter doing an exercise we call "good mornings": a standing motion in which you bend forward at the hip with straight legs with the weighted bar cupped behind the neck. Suddenly, the electric bolt shot through me during a rep; the weights went crashing and so did I. Only this time, I wasn't able to pop back up and that electrical sensation that usually came and quickly went . . . stayed. My lifting partner, Frank, had to pick me up off the floor.

I went to an imaging center for an MRI of my neck. I had put off any sort of procedure with my neck other than physical therapy to this point, partly because of my first experience with an MRI. Back when I was trying to earn a tryout with the Chiefs and weighing in at about 255 pounds, I was placed in one of the first

MRI tubes in Miami at Miami Children's Hospital. They shoehorned me into a tube that was designed for children and I remained in there for four hours. My chest and arms were pressed against the tube walls and my nose was pressed into the side of the tube. I should add that I'm claustrophobic. At the point when I was told there were thirty minutes remaining to complete the MRI, I informed the technician that I had had enough and to get me out of the tube. He replied "no" and said I needed to stay for the remaining thirty minutes, attempting to cheer me on while refusing to let me out. I told the technician in language I won't print here that when I got out of the tube, he had better not be within several miles of the hospital. Strike three—my confidence in surgical medicine was shot.

As I was exiting the imaging center in my scrubs on my way back to work, a man came running out of the building and asked me if I was Dr. McClain.

"Yes," I said with a hint of sarcasm I couldn't help, "how did you guess?"

He told me he was also a doctor and added, "I just read your MRI of your cervical spine. I have to tell you, I see a lot of these and most of them are kinda 50/50 as to there being anything recognizable or significant, but not yours. Do you know what you have going on here?"

Big pause from me while I let it sink in and remembered the last thirty-three years. "Well, I know I have a little something going on in my neck, obviously . . ."

"You have impingement on at least twenty-five percent of your spinal cord and myelomalacia [inflammation and edema—swelling of the spinal cord] and yet you don't have any symptoms?"

"Yeah, that's why I am here. Thanks for letting me know."

My next stop was to a neurosurgeon who told me that what I had was serious, and that while I might have some residual symptoms, he could "fix it." I asked if he could "fix it" at the end of the year in December (it was April at the time).

"Sure, but you won't be very happy waiting."

"Well, when do you recommend I take care of this?"

"Yesterday," he answered.

As of this writing, I have undergone more surgeries than I care to count—I stopped after twenty, but I imagine that I'm likely at about thirty or so—and that does not include procedures, which are considered more minor than surgery. I had the surgery he advised—within a day—and many more, and while the impingement to the spinal cord was relieved, the damage to the spinal cord (about 25 percent of the spinal cord, between C4 and C6) remains. As of this writing, I have artificial discs or fusions in approximately one-third of my vertebrae.

I have artificial right and left hips and—on the advice of my surgeon and shoulder replacement expert, John Itamura—I am waiting on the latest and greatest shoulder prostheses to be introduced in the United States before proceeding with shoulder replacements. I have had nerves rerouted and cut out, atrial fibrillation and atrial flutter, prostate and skin cancer, small intestine bacterial overgrowth, bacterial meningitis—and this list isn't even complete! I also have allergies to just about *everything* (thanks, Mom).

But *here's the thing*: I am in better shape than most people my age, as confirmed by some of the biological aging tests available today. To quote one of my favorite country western singers, Toby Keith, "I ain't as good as I once was, but I am as good once as I ever was." My genetics, epigenetic alterations, and injuries have not defined my quality of life. My dramatic injuries, botched medical procedures, and age do not confine me. While I may not be what I once was at twenty or thirty years old—and who is, at sixty?—I have been able to take advantage of medical advancements that have kept me alive, reduced my suffering, and enabled me to feel, act, and look years younger than I am. I play tennis, box, lift weights, hike, ski, bicycle (my wife and I just climbed the famed Mont Ventoux—the toughest climb on the Tour de France)—you name it, and I am still doing it. My past health battles, ones I sometimes almost lost to Death, do not define my healthspan or longevity. Not in the least.

I've cheated Death in every sense of that term—death of the body, of my mobility, of my sex drive, of my energy, and more.

Death will always win in the end, of course, but cheating Death means you take control of extending how long and how well you play the game.

THE MORAL OF THE STORY

I tell this story not to impress you with my suffering, but to impress upon you how blessed I've been because of medical advances—whether considered traditional or alternative medicine—despite my experiences earlier in life. I am alive and well both because of great doctors and surgeons and because I've been open to a wide range of treatments. Looking back, I realize that if I had consulted with doctors earlier, I would have had more options. But I was not even aware that there *were* options, just as many of you may be unaware of your own options.

Today, we're seeing advances and even breakthroughs that can make a huge difference in your healthspan. From stem cells—including a type of stem cell called Muse cells that can foster astonishing healing from a variety of diseases and disorders—to utilizing artificial intelligence (AI) devices that can alert us to health problems before they spiral out of control, we're on the cusp of a healthcare revolution.

So, part of my purpose in writing this book is to provide information about the latest options for improving health and extending lifespan. You'll read about emerging supplements that can slow or reverse the aging process, the benefits of cryotherapy, how green tea extract and other remedies are considered natural cancer fighters, and much more. But I also want to motivate you to reassess your ability to do something about your health and to discover your ability to live not only longer but healthier.

By seeing all the options, many of which are not being presented by managed healthcare, you may be driven to reassess your current conditions and health-related goals. What's so exciting to me—and what I hope will be equally exciting to you—is that you can do a lot more than you thought to increase how long and how well you live. I hope to make you aware of the range of relatively accessible and easy-to-use treatments that exist and how effective they can be. With this information, you can increase the odds of living the life you want to live now and for years to come. That's what healthspan is all about.

BE AN INFORMED CONSUMER

Last, I would be remiss if I failed to raise a yellow flag about everything I'm about to tell you. As much as I believe in and have researched and used the treatments and procedures that I'm going to present in these pages, I know from experience that time alters our perspective on best practices and even "science" itself. In the early 1950s or 1960s, a study came out that linked coffee to cancer. News of this study spread and there was legitimate concern in some medical circles that coffee consumption could lead to cancer. With hindsight, we know this study was flawed. Researchers failed to ask study participants one key question about a behavior that was—at the time—linked to coffee drinkers: Do you smoke?

Sometimes, studies suggest absolute truths that are only partial truths. For instance, a number of studies have linked salt consumption to hypertension. The well-known DASH diet, promoted by the National Heart, Lung, and Blood Institute, prescribed a fruit–grain–vegetable regimen with little or no added salt. We've learned, however, that excluding salt from your diet can be bad, that salt is especially essential for sweaty athletes, and that it does not necessarily lead to hypertension—at least for a significant number of people. Perhaps more surprising, it's been shown that excessive consumption of fructose (the predominant sugar in fruit) can promote hypertension and other diseases.

Even rigorous scientific studies are vulnerable to bias. Sometimes they're participant biases. Investigators ask participants questions and they respond with answers that they think are truthful, but often reflect unconscious bias. For instance, in a study of diet and obesity, participants may unknowingly exaggerate the amount of chocolate milk they consumed as children, since they're convinced that drinking all that chocolate milk is why they became fat.

The scientists, too, may be guilty of bias. Sometimes it's unconscious, as in the previous participant example, but sometimes they skew results based on their beliefs or because they have specific objectives. You may also be aware of research indicating that dietary restriction is the key to longevity. One meta-analysis (in effect, a study of several studies' results) examined a number of other studies on the subject and concluded that limiting what you eat can lead to a longer life. It turned out that the lead investigators cherry-picked the data that served their purposes and excluded data that didn't.

Unfortunately, most studies we reference—particularly those evaluating nutrition—are epidemiological, retrospective, and fraught with their accompanying severe limitations. That said, *some* of these studies have given us good leads to follow up on with more robust studies, and often, because of practical limitations, they are all we have to depend upon for insights. For a very comprehensive presentation regarding bias and study design, I recommend the five-part series "Studying Studies" by Peter Attia, MD,[1] and "Why Most Published Research Findings Are False" by John Ioannidis, MD.[2]

I have attempted to provide the latest information about every medication, supplement, procedure, and device that I discuss, and I've indicated when I feel more research is needed or if there are any risks involved. Nonetheless, things change quickly in the healthspan world—new studies, innovative methods, and products seem to surface daily. I ask you to view this book as a starting point for an improved lifespan, one that involves you in an ongoing discussion about regenerative possibilities and the evolving field of healthspan science, and I encourage you to talk to your doctor and do your own research before you try any treatment discussed here.

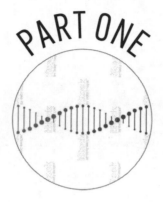

Regenerating Bodies, Rethinking Aging

Longevity Is the New Normal

BEFORE DELVING INTO specific healthspan-related treatments, let's frame them within a larger context—that of aging and regenerative medicine. Without this context, it might seem like some of these breakthrough approaches have emerged out of nowhere; some enterprising experimenter got lucky in the lab or, even worse, that they aren't grounded in valid research and scientific theory.

In fact, the treatments I'll detail are the product of extensive clinical studies, both in the US and other countries. Those of us in the field of regenerative medicine have spent many years examining the research or are involved with the research ourselves. We're aware not only of this research but of how it fits into theories of aging. Therefore, when we suggest a patient use cryotherapy to relieve arthritis pain or rely on peptides to restore their skin's youthful appearance, we're drawing on more than our empirical knowledge—we're taking advantage of the work of many scientists who have shared their data and conclusions.

To help you take advantage of their work, too, let's start out on a hopeful note—how, over time, aging has become something we're learning to control rather than letting it control us.

THE NATURE OF AGING

Years ago, many people didn't live past forty or fifty, perishing from a combination of poor nutrition and diseases without cures or even viable treatments. Today, our life expectancy is much longer—at least in the US, Europe, and other countries with access to good medical care. In the past, different types of bacteria were the leading cause of death. Dr. Alexander Fleming's discovery of penicillin was a game changer. As we developed more and more effective antibiotics, diseases that used to kill people became manageable, at least in the vast majority of cases.

Today, we often die from self-inflicted means. Certainly, some people die from things outside of their control—drunk drivers, genetically inherited diseases, and so on—but being obese, having poor nutrition, failing to get sufficient sleep, smoking and drinking to excess, getting no exercise, neglecting dental health, and too much sun all are behaviors that we know can kill us prematurely.

Our behaviors can increase or decrease the odds of how soon Death wins out. Heart disease is often manageable through exercise, diet, and medications. We've learned, too, that cancers don't just happen, but have environmental and other causes. We've also identified the causes or contributing factors that lead to diabetes, influenza, kidney disease, and many other maladies. Not only can we figure out the causes, but in a growing number of cases, we can manage the outcomes. Unlike the past, when heart disease, cancer, and diabetes were early death sentences, we've discovered ways to live with these ailments—or at least live longer and better than we did years ago.

We can't yet cure all cancer and some other diseases, but we now possess strategies to prevent some and control others. While aging isn't preventable, it is controllable—a radical shift from the traditional perspective that aging was inevitable and there was no point in fighting it. Dylan Thomas made famous a poem, "Do Not Go Gentle into That Good Night," one in which he urges us to "rage, rage against the dying of the light."

Aging is something that we can do something about; we need to get rid of our passive attitudes and be proactive in our responses to the passing of time. Our individual longevity used to be a game we had no control over; now we can rage against Death, in many cases cheating our way through extra years of vitality.

THE SIGNS OF AGING

While different theories have been proposed to explain why we age—theories that we'll discuss in the next section—scientists generally agree about the signs and symptoms of getting older. We know it's characterized by the following:

- immune function decline or dysfunction
- loss of muscle mass
- wrinkles
- gray hair
- decreased agility
- less strength and speed
- greater susceptibility to cancer, heart disease, and diabetes

Age is the most significant factor for many—if not most—diseases, which is why we start undergoing preventive diagnostic procedures such as colonoscopies as we become older.

Menopause and andropause happen to women and men, respectively, usually in their early fifties when sex hormones have already been decreasing for about fifteen years. As we get older, hearing and vision loss also may occur, as well as a gradual loss of muscle, often accompanied by a gradual gain of fat. Cognitive decline also may result as we become senior citizens.

Two general schools of thought have emerged about why these signs and symptoms of aging take place: predisposition (our biological parents, a.k.a. genetics) versus accumulation of damages due to environmental exposure to harmful substances and the choices we make. Certain forms of obesity are an example of the genetic-predisposition type, with some scientists pointing to genes that incline certain people to being overweight. An example of accumulation would be someone living next to a toxic-waste site for years who develops cancers associated with the poisons buried in the site after they leach into the groundwater. Some experts believe that it's the combination of accumulation and predisposition that produces the symptoms of aging—that a substantial component of aging is "predisposed," or genetically programmed to enable humans to evolve, and that our choices and "accumulation" of various insults to our health either accelerate that process or don't.

Furthermore, we still struggle with the definition of aging because we haven't been able to tease apart the diseases that accompany aging from the process of aging itself. For example, as we age—assuming we live long enough—our cognitive function begins to decline. Some of us need longer to calculate and become more forgetful; others, suffering from forms of dementia such as Alzheimer's disease, endure the devastating loss of most mental faculties. How much of the decline is due to aging and how much is due to a disease state such as Alzheimer's we have yet to determine, but it certainly appears that aging itself can predispose one to a multitude of diseases.

We're also not lacking in anti-aging treatments that range from scientifically valid to fraudulent. Some are variations of folk wisdom—"an apple a day keeps the doctor away" translates into eating lots of fruits and vegetables for a long, healthy life. Some are counterintuitive—one that received a lot of media attention in recent years was caloric restriction. In studies involving nonhuman organisms, limiting calories consumed to about 70 percent of normal levels has resulted in increased longevity. Other studies, however, reveal that caloric restriction not only fails to affect certain markers for aging positively but actually affects some of them negatively.

In the regenerative medicine community, we've developed numerous effective approaches that have been rigorously studied and tested—approaches that will be discussed throughout this book—but we've also discovered that one size doesn't fit all. We've learned that a treatment that works for one person may not work for another. We're all made slightly differently and these slight differences can have a huge impact on whether a given medication or procedure works for us. Consider that if you give amphetamines to some people, they'll become highly energized and active. But if you give these same amphetamines to people with attention-deficit/hyperactivity disorder—particularly in excess—they'll often respond by growing tired or actually falling asleep.

Individual differences matter not just in drug prescription effects, but also in aging. It takes a bit of experimentation to discover what works for you.

THEORIES OF HOW AND WHY WE AGE

As of this writing, there are nine generally accepted hallmarks of aging. They can be described slightly differently, but semantics aside, they generally fall into these categories:

1. **Genomic Instability**

   Genomic instability refers to a high frequency of mutations within the genome of a cellular lineage. Mutations can include changes in nucleic acid sequences, chromosomal rearrangements, or aneuploidy.

2. **Telomere Attrition**

   A reduction in the number of telomeres, which are the ends of mammalian chromosomes that form protective complexes that, together with telomerase (a specialized telomere-synthesizing enzyme), regulate telomere length.

3. **Epigenetic Alterations**

   Epigenetic changes alter the chemical structure of DNA, affecting its function without modifying its sequence.

4. **Deregulated Nutrient Sensing**

   Multiple nutrient sensing pathways are used to regulate intake and use of nutrients including mTOR, sirtuin, insulin and IGF-1, and AMPK. Deterioration of cellular function begins when these pathways become deregulated.

5. **Mitochondrial Dysfunction**

   A state of inefficient energy production resulting from damage to energy-producing cellular organelles called mitochondria.

6. **Cellular Senescence**

   A phenomenon characterized by cellular dysfunction and the cessation of cell division.

7. **Stem Cell Exhaustion**

   The age-related deficiency of stem cells. This particular hallmark is directly responsible for many of the physical problems associated with aging, such as frailty and a weakened immune system.

8. **Altered Intercellular Communication**[3]

   Dysregulated neurohormonal signaling between cells leading to cellular dysfunction.

9. **Loss of Proteostasis**
   Various proteins are created within the cell for specific functions, but occasionally some are not created properly, "misfolded" or not "folded," and thus must be corrected by refolding mechanisms or simply destroyed and/or recycled in the cell. Aggregations of nonfunctional proteins contribute to the dysfunction of the cell and "aging."

CELL SIGNALING

Research is being conducted into how this cellular-level communication system operates. We're finding that a given cell signal may be responsible for a number of regulatory and communication functions. Exosomes play a key role in cell signaling, and by studying them, we may better understand their role in spreading cancer cell to cell. More importantly, we may find ways to control this signaling and mitigate this spread.

While a number of explanations exist for aging, they often overlap in certain areas that can become scientifically granular. I'm not going to go too far down in the weeds in my discussions of these theories, but I do need to penetrate to the cellular level, since that's where a lot of the aging "aha!"s exist. Once you understand the different cellular processes affected by aging, you'll understand why there are so many pathways to restoring these processes to their original effectiveness. Let's start out with the free-radical theory of aging, one that goes hand in hand with the reactive oxygen species theory. Free radicals are molecules with an uneven number of electrons. The free radical theory of aging posits that molecules that have lost electrons can replace them by taking them from other molecules that make up the body's cells, often a destructive process. We create free radicals in our mitochondria—the powerhouse energy source of cells—when they convert food into usable energy. Free radicals, therefore, are part of a natural, essential process. After they're created, however, some avoid the cellular mechanisms designed to stop their reactivity and they end up disrupting cell signaling and functioning via processes we call oxidation (where one molecule loses one or more electrons) and reduction (where one molecule gains one or more electrons). Oxidation creates rust out of iron and the equivalent of rust in humans. Free radicals break down products from their original state and can impede normal cellular function, resulting in premature aging. Essentially, if we live long enough, we'll rust out.

The term *reactive oxygen species* includes free radicals (as well as non-free radicals), and while being essential for cells to do their jobs, it is this oxygen referenced within this terminology that is associated with neurodegenerative disorders, cancer, diabetes, and premature aging. It turns out that, like in so many things, the poison is in the dose. With certain therapies delivered in acutely stimulating doses—such as intravenous high-dose (typically more than 10 g) vitamin C, hyperbaric oxygen therapy, and ozone therapy—reactive oxygen species can be very beneficial. One way to think about it is if, like Robin Hood, you're robbing the rich to provide for the suffering poor. When you've robbed all the rich, you don't want to begin robbing good citizens, but if you have some other "bad" citizens—like cancer, for example—that aren't necessarily rich, but need to be stopped regardless, you do actually want to rob them, too.

This dovetails with two related theories of aging—mitochondrial dysfunction and mutation—that attribute the aging process to overproduction or mismanagement of naturally occurring reactive oxygen species. When reactive oxygen species are created, but aren't used by cells, they can cause damage that can age us prematurely. Though mitochondria making usable energy from food is an essential process, the excessive oxidation that can result is why we get wrinkles, lose muscle, have decreased immune function, and so on. Mitochondria are also energy-producing components (organelles) of your cells essential for hormonal signaling, cellular repair, heartbeat (muscular contraction), and protecting DNA integrity. Given these wide-ranging tasks, mitochondrial function also plays a determinative role in sexual health.

To use a simple example, we all know that a certain amount of exercise is good for us. We promote our *health* best—not necessarily our *athletic* best—by exercising enough to stimulate many processes that keep us functioning at our peak, but not by exercising *too* much, going beyond our body's ability to recover and/or to recover without sacrificing one area of health for another.

Fortunately, several scientists now believe that methods exist to reverse or at least control this process; that we can limit the amount of oxidation that occurs or even possibly repair the damage it causes. Throughout the book, I will examine these methods and show how they can take advantage of our natural cell-repair capabilities.

Another theory of aging is cellular senescence: the condition in which the cell can no longer reproduce by dividing, yet remains metabolically but dysfunctionally active. This theory holds that over time, DNA damage to the cell accumulates and leads to cell malfunction and concomitant problems with related organs. Dysfunctioning cells wreak havoc within themselves and upon other cells. Think of it as an engine that is still running but, because it can no longer be tuned, is spewing poisonous exhaust fumes and polluting its surroundings. David Sinclair, a biologist and professor at Harvard Medical School and author of *Lifespan: Why We Age—and Why We Don't Have To*, employs a different analogy to describe cellular senescence: a damaged CD that no longer plays right. The coding—the information akin to DNA within the CD—has been corrupted through one of several ways, from reactive oxygen species to problems with our natural cellular repair system to radiation exposure. When cells aren't working properly, the damage spreads and leads to aging-related issues. When free radicals damage the mitochondria or the whole cell, these corrupted structures can't function or replicate effectively. When we can't replace our dysfunctioning essential parts, we stop forming healthy new cells that fight against diseases, keep our heart beating healthfully, and regulate how we process the sugar in our blood. In short, we age.

Yet another theory of aging is related to cellular senescence, but involves other regulatory mechanisms that produce cell-signaling breakdown and dysfunction. Early on, for most of us, cells do well on their own. In fact, our bodies naturally rid us of bad cells through a process called autophagy, a natural cellular repair process that clears out damaged cells while replicating healthy cells to replace them. For instance, proteins get broken down for many reasons and, when they're "misfolded" within the cell, that cell begins working improperly, so our cells try to rid themselves of these dysfunctional proteins through autophagy. When the proteins can't be eliminated, they float around and cause damage that promotes various diseases and, again, can make us age prematurely. We find we can't carry as much weight, can't walk as fast, or aren't as agile as we once were, and the problems can multiply. Oversensitivity or insensitivity to insulin can cause cellular breakdowns. An overly robust immune system response is another issue; when this response occurs, it attacks what are actually well-functioning systems within the body; the autoimmune disease lupus is an example.

When we talk about proteins and aging, we must look at the mTOR gene, named for the mammalian or mechanistic target of rapamycin. The protein it encodes, also called mTOR, is a signaling protein and, as such, it can foster cell replication. While growth can be a good thing, it can become a problem as we become older—the growth of cancer cells, for instance. Too much mTOR can fuel cancer and excessive insulin production. Essentially, mTOR can create too many "bad" cells, and its engagement prevents other important processes such as autophagy from occurring. Later in the book we'll discuss rapamycin, a drug that can reduce the function of mTOR.

Telomere shortening fits in this cellular senescence category as well. Telomeres are structures at the ends of chromosomes that shorten over time. They reflect the number of divisions remaining in a cell. As they shorten, the cell approaches its division limit and eventually dies. They protect this portion of the chromosome, similar to the way a plastic cap (aglet) protects the end of a shoelace. Over time, the telomeres become shorter and less protective. Imagine the way a shoelace unravels when its cap falls apart and you'll get the picture. When chromosomal DNA unravels, holds the theory, we age. Shortened telomeres rob cells of their ability to function properly and replicate. All this makes us vulnerable to various diseases, including heart disease and cancer. It's also been suggested that free radicals contribute to telomere shortening, so, again, we believe there is much crossover between the theories of aging and how they operate.

DNA methylation is a natural and beneficial process that regulates genetic expression, but the theory is that abnormal DNA methylation can occur and produce the effects of aging. Methylation can turn genes on and off, and scientists have found that some people are genetically predisposed to live longer—or, at the other end of the spectrum, to be prone to certain diseases. Abnormal DNA methylation makes us more vulnerable to these diseases, though the hope is that gene editing can address this issue. DNA methylation theory provides an aging measurement, helping us assess biological or "real" age versus chronological age. This is a reflection of cellular aging and suggests that certain genes and their epigenetic expression (i.e., environmentally stimulated changes to genes, rather than alteration of underlying hereditary genetic code) influence our real age.

Yet another theory of aging revolves around advanced glycation end products (AGEs), which are considered biomarkers of aging. These products occur when fats or proteins combine with sugars; they occur naturally in various foods, but certain cooking methods can increase their content. They are crosslinks between sugars and either proteins or lipids (fats) and can lead to degenerative diseases such as Alzheimer's, coronary artery disease (CAD), and diabetes. AGEs are known to accelerate the aging process and are associated with oxidative stress and inflammation.

The inflammation AGEs produce cause intercellular damage and cell death. A significant amount of research is being conducted on how to prevent AGEs from having these negative effects.

AGES AND GLUCOSEPANE

Glucosepane is the most common AGE, and Revel is one company that is working to create enzymes that target and counter glucosepane. This could mean that we'll be able to restore blood vessels and skin flexibility, reversing stiffness and preventing the concomitant diseases of aging.

Besides these theories, a number of others exist that help explain why we age. Nuclear factor kappa B, for instance, helps explain how excessive inflammation leads to diabetes, cancer, and arthritis. Other theories exist, and scientists have different names and categories for these theories. We're still developing a consistent and comprehensive theory of aging and, until we do so, some confusion and uncertainty about how and why our bodies deteriorate over time will exist. Nonetheless, it's still important to be aware of the major theories, since they have become the basis for a number of effective treatments. For anyone interested in living longer, healing faster, and looking better, these theories offer scientific evidence for a range of products and procedures that we'll discuss. As you'll see, these theories have inspired many studies and have helped regenerative medicine specialists develop effective approaches.

PUTTING THEORIES INTO PRACTICE

As researchers have explored theories about aging, they've learned a lot about cellular functioning in general and about a specific type of cell in particular—stem cells. These are chameleon-like cells that are capable of differentiating into cells with specialized functions: brain cells, heart muscle cells, and so on. We've learned how to use these stem cells in laboratories by removing them from patients, differentiating them in the lab, and then injecting them back into patients. These stem cells can be used to regenerate diseased and damaged tissue and have been used effectively here and in other countries to treat a range of conditions, from osteoarthritis to spinal cord injuries.

I don't want to describe specific stem cell therapies here, but I do want to share two stories that illustrate how the study of aging has yielded breakthrough results for patients.

David Lyons was a middle-aged man who had been diagnosed with multiple sclerosis (MS) and who began receiving stem cell therapy in 2014. David was my patient, and he had told me that he was going to receive this therapy from a company called American CryoStem in the Cayman Islands; he was the first American CryoStem patient to receive this type of treatment for MS. They started him on a small amount of stem cells (fifty million) the first day, delivered over the course of an hour for safety reasons. He did fine, so the next day, they increased the dose to a hundred million cells.

David experienced remarkable improvements in his vision, gait, and strength without any adverse effects. I was so impressed with the strides he made that I contacted the head of American CryoStem and eventually became a member of their medical and scientific advisory board, as well as an investigator in its research study to gain FDA approval of stem cell use in the US as an Investigational New Drug (IND). Subsequently, David received additional treatments from other providers that have also been successful. He recounted his amazing recovery from the worst symptoms of multiple sclerosis in an online article.[4]

Another patient of mine, a young woman named Judy, was suffering from aggressive Crohn's disease, an inflammatory disorder in which the immune system attacks itself and causes a number of unpleasant, painful intestinal symptoms. When Judy came to us, she was taking prednisone and a high-dose form of aspirin. Prednisone can have nasty side effects, including insomnia and bloating, and we switched her off these medications and started her on L-glutamine, an amino acid that helps synthesize and repair tissue and can facilitate gut health without the negative side effects of stronger medications. We also had Judy take enteric-coated peppermint oil capsules to soothe the gut and reduce inflammation. While this approach helped Judy control her disease, it didn't cure it.

That's when we turned to stem cells. We harvested her own stem cells and then infused them back into her body. Within months, all of Judy's symptoms resolved. Now we give her an infusion of stem cells once or twice yearly to control the disease and she continues to do well without having to take the strong medications traditionally used to treat Crohn's. We speculate that, as with other autoimmune disorders, if we could treat her with a larger amount of stem cells, it's possible that the overwhelming dose would recalibrate her immune system and cure the disease altogether. Judy then wouldn't require additional maintenance stem cell infusions. However, regulatory issues and practical considerations prohibit us from giving her this larger amount. I'll address the regulatory issues in later chapters.

What I hope you take away from these two brief stories is that both patients suffered from degeneration and stem cell treatments provided regeneration. Regenerative therapy in various forms is the wave of the future and we need more people—patients, doctors, and researchers—to recognize what's coming and learn more about it.

NOT JUST LIVING LONGER, BUT LIVING BETTER

When people of a certain age complain to their doctors about various aches and pains, insomnia, sexual performance, and not having their former energy, doctors often respond by saying words to the effect of, "You have to learn to live with it," and, "It's just a normal part of aging." The typical medical view has been that people should accept the deterioration that comes with age as natural, that it's vain to want to erase wrinkles and even somewhat presumptuous to fight a battle that they can't win.

While there is no panacea for aging (yet), there are viable regenerative options and it's irrational not to avail yourself of them. For instance, the first aging theory we discussed was the free radical theory. We are learning how to use antioxidants to get rid of excess free radicals and reactive oxygen species. If we can find the right balance of antioxidants, we can limit the damage done and slow the aging process. This isn't a pipe dream. Antioxidant therapy is easily available and affordable. Though we're still trying to find the right balance of antioxidants for individual patients, they are still a potent weapon in the fight against aging. Thus, before you go out to purchase a bag of antioxidants, know that you, too, must strike a balance between antioxidants and free radicals; too many antioxidants can be a bad thing. Remember, reactive oxygen species can actually be beneficial in small and/or acute doses. For more on this, I recommend the book *Guilty Until Proven Innocent: Antioxidants, Foods, Supplements, and Cosmetics* written by a brilliant chemist and my friend, Dr. Gagik Melikyan.

Ultimately, it's not just about living longer. Who wants to live to be a hundred if the last twenty years of life are spent bedridden and in pain? Healthspan is the key. It's quality of life, not just quantity. In fact, if you ask most patients (and their doctors) if they would be willing to trade quantity for quality in their own lives, most would answer affirmatively. In the healthspan community, there's a term: "squaring the curve." Imagine a piece of paper with health on the vertical axis and age on the horizontal one.

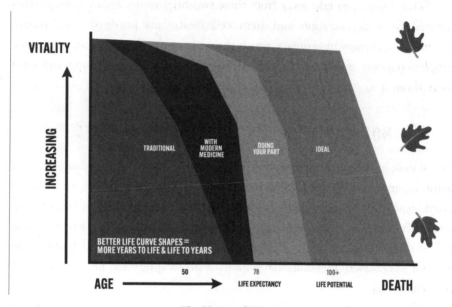

VITALITY

INCREASING

TRADITIONAL

WITH MODERN MEDICINE

DOING YOUR PART

IDEAL

BETTER LIFE CURVE SHAPES = MORE YEARS TO LIFE & LIFE TO YEARS

AGE

50

78
LIFE EXPECTANCY

100+
LIFE POTENTIAL

DEATH

The "Squared" Curve

If we draw a line tracing our health and age on this page, it usually starts out high when we're young but curves precipitously downward during our final decades on the planet. Healthspan's goal is to straighten that line so that it remains straight and high, creating a square on the page.

This book is designed in part as a guide to healthspan-friendly practices (ways to cheat Death), offering a variety of tools that can help you improve your physical fitness, diminish the outward signs of aging, recover faster from injury, restore youthful vim and vigor, prevent or identify early diseases that can age us prematurely, and achieve many other beneficial objectives.

AGE IS RELATIVE

As the saying goes, "It doesn't matter how old you are; it's how you feel that counts." Age really is just a number. One sixty-year-old male is engaging in vigorous daily gym workouts, looks like he's fifty, and is having sex with his wife three times a week. Another sixty-year-old is out of breath just walking around the block, looks like he's seventy, and hasn't had sex in the last two years.

Consider chronological versus biological age. The former reflects your age in years lived, the latter reflects your relative physical health. I probably don't need to point out that the two ages often are quite different. I've found that people need a self-assessment tool, one that can help them determine their biological age and whether there's a gap with their chronological age. If the gap is positive—their chronological age is higher than their biological age—then this tool can reinforce all the positive behaviors they've adopted to keep themselves in good shape. If the gap is negative, then it serves as motivation to give up bad habits and do the things necessary to be biologically younger than their chronological age.

There's a lot you can do to close a negative gap and open up a positive one. Some are obvious—get more sleep, stop smoking, eat more nutritious food. A lot of changes, however, aren't obvious. For instance, most people don't realize that you can tailor your diet to encourage autophagy—the natural cell repair process discussed in further detail in chapters six and thirteen—or that cryotherapy is an astonishingly effective method for reducing arthritis pain.

Working with other healthcare professionals, I'm in the process of developing a method to calculate biological age. It's still in its relative infancy, but is based on multiple measurable factors and is remarkably accurate, beginning with just these sixteen:

- date of birth
- gender
- height and weight
- ethnic heritage
- state where you've lived the longest
- calorie intake
- exercise amount
- sleep amount
- laboratory assays: HbA1C, fasting insulin, vitamin D3, neutrophil-to-lymphocyte ratio, CRP, testosterone, VO_2 max

These aren't the only factors that help make a biological age calculation—other blood tests and assays are also important to adjusting the calculation—but they can provide a relatively accurate assessment. Once we've made this assessment, we're in a much better position to know what steps we need to take to improve our healthspan as well as our longevity.

For our purposes here, you can do a very rough estimate of your biological age by determining your BMI (from height and weight), looking up your expected lifespan (based on your gender, ethnicity, and state), estimating your calories consumed (and where that number falls versus the recommended amount for your age, gender, and height), and figuring out if you get the recommended amount of exercise.

Even if you don't want to go to the trouble of doing this calculation, you probably have a good sense of your health relative to some of these factors; you are aware of whether you overeat, don't get any or sufficient exercise, are overweight, or are not getting enough sleep.

The good news is that when it comes to extending the healthspan game, most of us have numerous options for slowing down or turning back the chronological clocks. The following chapters will describe these options (cheats) in detail.

2

Measuring Biological Versus Chronological Age

Telomeres and Methylation

LIVING LONGER AND feeling and looking better is a healthspan dream. This dream is closer than ever to reality because of our growing understanding of telomeres and methylation. Let's start out with definitions, since these terms may not be familiar to everyone.

Every cell in your body carries a set of genes that is unique to you; the genes tell the cell what to do and when to do it. These genes, composed of DNA, are linked together in long strands called chromosomes with twenty-three pairs of chromosomes in each cell. At the end of each chromosome is a protective cap called a telomere; it protects the chromosome from being damaged when the cell divides. Composed of thousands of sections of "expendable DNA," telomeres shorten slightly each time a cell divides. An abundance of shortened telomeres has been linked to premature aging and disease.

Perhaps one analogy to telomeres that may be apropos is to think of them like years of warranty. The longer the telomere, the more cell divisions—free replacements under warranty—that can occur.

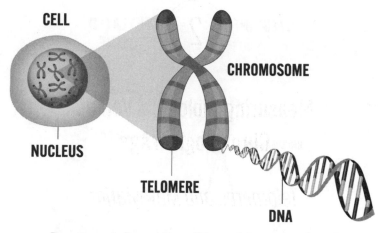

CELL

CHROMOSOME

NUCLEUS

TELOMERE

DNA

Diagrammatic Perspective on Telomeres's Presence in the Cell

DNA methylation is the biological process by which a methyl group (a carbon molecule with three hydrogens attached to it) is added to DNA molecules. By bonding with the cytosine (one of the four nucleotides present in DNA) component of DNA, it can modify how genes function (without altering gene sequences), which can have a significant impact on longevity as well as various diseases. The term *epigenetics* is crucial for understanding this impact. The epigenome is defined as changes in gene activity that are not caused by changes in DNA sequence. The epigenetic effect of DNA methylation is so significant because it means that you don't have to be resigned to the genetic cards you're dealt at birth. You may have DNA that predisposes you to various disorders and diseases, but the DNA methylation process can be used diagnostically, as well as manipulated through healthspan-promoting methods outlined in this book, to promote healing. To return to our analogy, it helps prevent the harmful cards in your hand from being played.

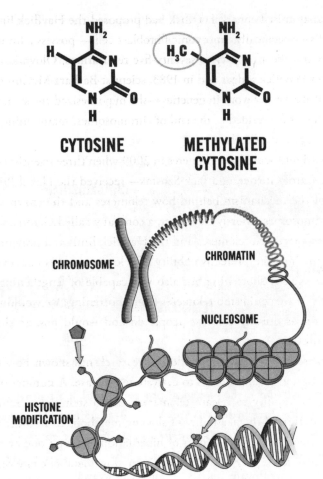

Diagrammatic Presentation of Where DNA Methylation Occurs

With these basic definitions out of the way, let's examine both these topics from a healthspan perspective.

LONGER IS BETTER... USUALLY

Let's put telomeres in a historical scientific context—one that helps explain the importance of telomeres to longevity.

Alexey Olovnikov is the Russian scientist who, in 1971, first identified the problem of telomere shortening and how it was related to aging. Earlier, the

American anatomist Leonard Hayflick had proposed the Hayflick limit, suggesting that cells—specifically, embryonic fibroblast cells—possess a limited capacity for division and die after fifty to seventy-five replications. Olovnikov and others expanded on Hayflick's ideas and in 1983, scientist Barbara McClintock received the Nobel Prize for her work in genetics—she hypothesized the structure of telomeres and how they resided at the end of chromosomes, maintaining their structure like the aglet of a shoelace.

The spotlight focused on telomeres in 2009 when three scientists—Elizabeth Blackburn, Carol Greider, and Jack Szostak—received the Nobel Prize for their discovery of the mechanism behind how telomeres and the enzyme telomerase protect chromosomes. Shortly thereafter, a company called Geron confirmed the link between shortened telomeres and the Hayflick limit and provided more scientific insight into the protective ability of telomerase; this enzyme could not only protect against shortening but also was capable of lengthening telomeres. Theoretically, if we could stop telomeres from shortening, we wouldn't reach the Hayflick limit as quickly as most people do and would possess the ability to extend our lifespan.

Since these discoveries, a great deal of research has shown how to use gene therapies, drugs, and supplements to activate telomerase. A number of chemicals demonstrate the ability to release telomerase, as do stem cells. Some scientists have also investigated the possibility of slowing metabolisms in order to slow cell divisions—essentially, this is a form of hibernation. Though one of my teachers used to tell us that the only way to achieve a very low metabolic rate was immobility in *very* cold environments, we may discover a drug that can slow our metabolisms without forcing us into a hibernating state. In fact, as will be mentioned later, there's evidence that metformin and berberine can improve metabolic function.

What good does it do us to know all this information about telomeres and telomerase? After all, it's not as if there's a surgical procedure that can lengthen all the telomere strands at the end of chromosomes and help us live longer.

While no surgical technique for this exists, this knowledge benefits us in two ways: (1) it serves as a warning sign relative to aging and disease, and (2) it gives us the opportunity to respond in ways that stop our telomeres from shortening and help us try to lengthen them.

We've learned that shortened telomeres reflect not only lifespan but also a variety of diseases including cardiovascular disease, type 2 diabetes, chronic obstructive pulmonary disorder, Alzheimer's, schizophrenia, arthritis, and cancer.

The last one is particularly interesting, in that short telomeres are indicative of cancer, but once the cancer is established, it thrives based on its access to telomerase. Recall the subhead to this section—that longer is better *usually*—in that longer-than-normal telomere strands actually help cancer thrive.

My point: telomere length (or rather, lack thereof) can be a warning sign we need to heed. Telomeres can also be used for their predictive value. We can treat a disease and then test telomeres every six months to determine if they're continuing to shorten, if we've stopped the shortening process, or if they're growing longer. In this way, we can determine if our medical interventions for a given disease are working.

Telomeres can also work as a screening tool. If we observe unusually long telomeres, that can alert us to the presence of cancer before other tests or symptoms reveal it. Perhaps most obviously, telomeres can tell us our biological age versus our chronological age. We might be forty-eight years of age, but the shortened telomeres indicate our biological age is sixty-eight. Or the opposite may be true—we're sixty-eight, but the telomeres are healthfully long, suggesting our biological age is forty-eight. These results tell us that either we need to make changes or intervene in some way, or reassure us that we're in great shape.

TEST TO MEASURE YOUR TELOMERES

Three types of tests are available commercially to determine your telomere length. Let's look at the pros and cons of each:

- **qPCR.** This test has been around longer than most others and is relatively affordable; $100 is the typical cost. Some of the companies that offer this test also have a good database of results, and it may offer a generally accurate indication of telomere length. The problem, though, is that testing is done by extrapolating results from a small sample. Consequently, you can end up with false readings—if the sample size selected has a long telomere length, the test may extrapolate that the average length of all telomeres is this length. However, the tiny sample may not be representative of other telomeres.
- **Flow FISH.** This testing method combines flow cytometry with the counting and measuring of cells through a system called FISH (fluorescent in situ hybridization). Using a flow cytometer, it measures

fluorescence levels of cells that have been put through the FISH system. More accurate than the qPCR method, it's also more labor intensive and therefore more expensive. It provides both the mean (average) and the median (middle value) of the telomere lengths.

- **HT Q-FISH.** High-throughput quantitative FISH is the most accurate telomere test, extracting a greater sample size for the test through flow cytometry. Combining a microscope with fluorescence, it offers the mean (average) and median telomere lengths, as well as the percentage distribution of specific telomere lengths. This method helps identify telomeres that are critically short rather than just providing a mean or median telomere length. It can identify a quantity of telomeres in the body that are long versus how many are short. Mean or median numbers can hide the problem of overly short telomeres—the median or mean may be fine, but still fail to spotlight telomeres that can be problematic.

EASY METHODS FOR LENGTHENING YOUR TELOMERES

Once you've used one of these methods to assess your telomeres, you can take steps to restore or at least maintain their length. The good news is that these steps aren't expensive and don't require complex medical treatments or experimental procedures. Instead, research shows that you can stop telomeres from shortening and possibly lengthen them by adopting good health habits. Here are some suggestions:

- **Exercise regularly.** Reducing oxidative stress and preserving DNA through regular workouts is essential for keeping telomeres a decent length. Some research indicates that men in their fifties who exercise have the same-length telomeres as men in their twenties.
- **Keep your BMI low.** While BMI is not necessarily the best fitness measure (one can be well muscled, lean, and fit and have a relatively high BMI), being "big"—especially but not limited to having too much fat—can affect telomeres negatively. If you know any people in their eighties or nineties, you'll notice that very few of them are fat. And, even if lean and muscular, how many "big" older men and women do you know?
- **Eat a Mediterranean diet or its equivalent.** Some research suggests that diets rich in omega-3 fats, fewer saturated fats, and more plant-based foods can keep telomeres at healthy lengths. Still, this is an area where

the data isn't particularly strong (most diets are limited by strictly epidemiological studies), so it may be worthwhile to see what new studies reveal about this topic. The most important factor for diets' effect on telomere length is their effect on systemic inflammation. While this is a very general statement, it is also very likely applicable to almost any cellular process and biological age marker, since inflammation is the substance or protagonist that, when present in excess, "gums up the works" of most biology.

- *Use supplements.* Vitamin D3 is a good supplement to take and, in general, antioxidant supplements in moderation provide anti-aging assistance to our bodies. Conceivably, this assistance includes maintaining telomere length.

- *Reduce stress.* Studies show a link between prematurely shortened telomeres and stress. While stress reduction is challenging for many people, living longer is a compelling incentive to make the effort, whether that effort takes the form of meditation, long walks in the woods, or various relaxation-breathing techniques.

Other standard healthy-living recommendations—limit alcohol consumption, stop smoking, get help for depression—should all be part of a telomere-lengthening strategy.

USING TELOMERES AND DNA METHYLATION TO PREDICT DISEASE AND PROMOTE HEALTH

Earlier I explained the epigenetic role of methylation and that, though DNA remains the same, methylation can determine how the DNA is marked and activated (or not activated). In humans, methylation of DNA acts on cytosine, one of its four nucleotides (the sugar, nitrogen, and phosphate "building blocks" whose mutual bonds provide the structure of DNA or RNA), and affects how the genetic material binds. Conversely, reducing methylation suppresses the activity of certain genes.

Since the 1960s, researchers have seen a connection between DNA methylation and aging. Steve Horvath, a UCLA professor of human genetics and biostatistics, helped create an epigenetic clock in 2013 by relying on DNA methylation data from the cytosine nucleotide. Measuring methylated DNA collected from a drop of blood, Horvath's clock correlated positively 98 percent of the time with chronological age. A number of other studies also have linked DNA methylation, age, and age-related outcomes. While other models competitive to Horvath's clock have emerged, his is still the one most widely used.

The value of this measurement is that we can use that one-drop blood sample to determine if someone is aging slower or faster than is typical. The results can be compared with databases of DNA methylation tests of centenarians to see if they compare favorably. Combining these results with telomere testing, we can develop a good sense of an individual's potential for living longer. If this person is aging too quickly, we can launch efforts to slow the aging process.

If you're interested in measuring your age using DNA methylation, Horvath's clock became available commercially in 2019 from a company called Elysium Health, and its price was $500 when introduced.

Methylation testing can also be used to better understand other diseases and, along with other biomarkers, help identify diseases in people who don't know they have them. Why? Age is typically the biggest risk factor for the most prevalent diseases such as colon cancer, CAD, type 2 diabetes, and so forth. But this fact is rarely mentioned because heretofore, we have considered age as something we can't control. So, we focus on things we can do something about, such as sleep, exercise, and diet. When we use age as a screening factor, we base it on chronological age. Doesn't it make more sense to base these screenings on biological age (as well as other pertinent factors, such as first-degree relatives having the disease), so that, especially for an individual who is biologically older, these potentially life-saving screenings can be performed at more optimal times?

Scientists are now studying the link between DNA methylation and lupus, muscular dystrophy, and birth defects with the goal of using this testing to prevent or treat these diseases.

Perhaps the most promising use involves cancer. Drugs targeting DNA methylation have been approved by the FDA for treatment of various cancers and are now going through trials. Recall my earlier point that DNA methylation can suppress certain types of genetic activity. Tumor-suppressor genes are often silenced in cancer cells due to hypermethylation. To activate these genes, scientists are working on drugs that can reverse methylation.

For people who are primarily concerned with healthspan issues, though, there are a number of simple, inexpensive steps to take, similar to our earlier telomere-lengthening suggestions.

Again, exercise is great—we know it reduces methylation. Minimizing alcohol consumption also has the same effect. And a diet rich in omega-3 fats (fish and flaxseed oils) as well as fruits, vegetables, and poultry also has a reductive impact. Alpha-tocopherol, a form of vitamin E found in olive oil, likewise reduces methylation.

We also need to avoid foods and treat disorders and conditions that increase methylation. For instance, gamma-tocopherol, found in black walnuts, sesame seeds, pecans, and pistachios, raises methylation. So, too, do high insulin levels, decreased insulin sensitivity, high triglyceride levels, and high blood pressure. And again, having fat around the waist can lead to increased methylation.

Anti-aging medicine is advancing by leaps and bounds, and my goal here is not to cover every advance but rather to focus on telomeres and methylation, since they have great potential as diagnostic tools and healing methods.

3

Improving Healthspan with Intentional Nutrition

WHAT IF I told you that food is the most powerful drug you will ever take? While food is not typically classed as a pharmacological intervention, as you'll see, its potency rivals many drugs.

If we take a step back in time—say, about two million years or so—we have some fairly solid evidence from the anthropological record that our ancestors' increase in brain size came about as a result of a surplus in animal fats and proteins, via innovations in stone projectile weapons and group hunting of large animals. Once the use of fire increased the bioavailability of those fats and proteins, human brains became even larger. By modern times, we had acquired language faculty and we more or less had what we see now when we look in the mirror.

For at least the last 250,000 years, with some geographical variation, our primary food sources were animal meats, complemented by a modest intake of plant fibers and seasonal availability of fruits. About 10,000 years ago, however, a fairly significant change to human nutrition occurred: the advent of agriculture.

As we settled in one place to secure our food and increased our carbohydrate intake by growing large quantities of foods with a higher glycemic load, we improved our health and our longevity in that epoch.

How does any of this understanding help us make better choices about what we eat?

It suggests that just as we've made quantum nutritional leaps in the past, we can do so again today using our greater knowledge about the effect of different types of food on our bodies. My patients want to use food to look and feel better, and by extension, lower their risk for what I like to call the Five Deadly Scourges:

1. Obesity
2. Diabetes
3. Neurocognitive decline
4. Cardiac disease
5. Cancer

Fear of disease and death combined with a desire for improved cosmetic appearance and internal vitality are phenomenally motivating factors, helping people make more optimal choices when it comes to their daily nutrition.

HOW TO CHOOSE A GOOD NUTRITION PLAN OVER A FAD

Here's a trick question: What is the single best diet for everyone's health?

The answer: there is no such diet.

Nonetheless, the media creates a lot of buzz around different diets like the keto diet, the Mediterranean diet, and so on. Some of these diets are fine (though some are not), but they fail to take into account that *one size doesn't fit all*. The only diet that comes close to working for most people with CAD is Dr. Dean Ornish's diet—a low-saturated-fat, high-carb (largely vegetable) diet that slows, stops, and even reverses arterial plaque deposits. That aside, people need to tailor their diets to their genetics, specific diseases and disorders they're experiencing, and health-related goals—the test for metabolic health that I just described is especially useful. If you're an athlete and require muscle, you'll need more protein—not the Twinkies diet.

Beware of anyone who insists that "you" should be on a particular diet. As attractive as supposed diet panaceas are, it's extremely difficult to assess the value of most diets. Part of the problem is that it's difficult to do scientifically valid studies about diets—to put people in controlled environments and make sure they adhere to a strict regimen of food over a long period. That's why most studies are done through interviewing participants and noting their recollections of what they consumed. But people's memories are often unreliable. On top of this, it's difficult to control the quality of food—one person is eating organic salmon, another farm-raised fish, a third freshly caught.

In addition, some studies and scientists demonize a particular food group. Instead of insisting that a particular diet is good for anyone, these naysayers insist that a particular food is bad for everyone. Sugar, for instance, has been attacked for numerous reasons—perhaps good reasons. But I've also seen more than one race won because of the burst of energy sugar provides. Gatorade, the drink of athletes, is composed primarily of sugar and electrolytes, and it (or its many variations) has helped many athletes on race or training day. But it is the person—athlete or not—who sips Gatorade or its sugary equivalent at every meal (or in place of a meal) that suffers the ill effects of excess sugar and gives it a bad name. And there's the more existential issue of whether you want to live life without some sweetness. I'd suggest that an occasional donut or piece of cake is good for the soul. That said, we are using some sugar substitutes such as allulose, erythritol, and stevia in foods and beverages that sweetly affect the soul without harming the rest of us like excess sugar does.

To find the right diet for your particular circumstances, do the following:

- Begin by making an appointment with a registered dietician or nutritionist who possesses experience advising people about the effect of diet on the body. Be aware that some of these dieticians and nutritionists will follow the standard American diet ("SAD") guidelines, which may not be optimal for your particular needs. Ideally, you'll find someone who can help you tailor your diet to your particular nutritional goals.
- Determine your goals for your diet. Do you want to be able to run a marathon, reduce LDL cholesterol, or protect yourself against a genetic disease to which you're vulnerable?
- Find a diet that fits your age. Our bodies work differently as we grow older, and our nutritional requirements change. For instance, as we age, we may make less vitamin D, lose more calcium, and absorb less iron and other nutrients. Therefore, older people will need to replace these important nutrients through diet and/or supplementation.
- Tailor your diet to your current health situation. Are you overweight? Do you have a particular disease or disorder? Do you lack energy?

Perhaps the best advice is to use the trial-and-error method. Figure out what diet works best for you by asking yourself regularly: How do I look? How do I feel? How do I perform? Keep a food journal to note how what you eat seems to be affecting you in these three ways. Do it for a month or so and test different diets. Admittedly, this isn't the most scientific method, but sometimes empirical methods provide insights that science can't.

ADD B VITAMINS TO ALL FOOD PLANS

Deficiencies of B vitamins can cause significant health risks. We use up these "stress" vitamins quickly, and therefore need to supplement them above and beyond our nutritional plan. B vitamins convert food into energy through the citric acid cycle (also known as the Krebs cycle), so they are key to our energy levels. They also serve other purposes, such as promoting cell health and brain function. To supplement, look for B-complex products—they contain the full range of B vitamins. They can take a while to work, and because these vitamins are water soluble, they aren't easily stored. People who consume sufficient amounts of meat (meats include sources from all animals), eggs, leafy green vegetables, dairy, and seeds are usually not as B deficient, but I rarely see individuals replete in sufficient B vitamins unless supplementing. While B-complex products are recommended, bioavailability varies—some B-vitamin products aren't as well absorbed as others. Ask your doctor, nutritionist, or pharmacist for recommendations.

Scientific monitoring is particularly appropriate for certain people. A blood test may reveal you're deficient in calcium or that you have diabetes or prediabetes, and this knowledge—especially when used with other monitoring devices (e.g., a continuous blood glucose monitor for diabetes)—can help you adjust your diet accordingly. Similarly, if you have high blood pressure, you may want to adjust your mineral intake or influence any fluid-retaining hormones. Or, if a coronary CT angiogram reveals arterial plaque, you may want to reduce your consumption of saturated fats.

Even the "right" diet, though, sometimes can't remedy problems that are a result of less controllable factors, such as genetics or viral or bacterial infections, which can seed inflammation in the coronary arteries and lead to plaque formation. I've had patients in my practice who are great athletes but who, upon having an angiogram, discovered a 99 percent blockage in their left anterior descending artery—the cause of "widowmaker" heart attacks—and they needed stents to clear blockages. Many times, physical fitness or diet doesn't overcome a bad genetic hand or poor dental hygiene—you can be in great shape but still be vulnerable to heart problems or diabetes. Conversely, some people are blessed with great genetics; I know individuals who eat what many cardiologists would consider terrible diets but whose arteries are free of plaque.

CUSTOM PLANNED FOOD PROGRAMS

The tough part is getting started. A broad array of easily accessible and highly palatable foods tempts us and a deluge of competing, often contradictory information about what the "best" diet is confuses us.

A good beginning point is working backward from what patients' goals are. Sometimes they are modest: "Hey, I just want to be able to fit into my wedding dress again." Often, they are ambitious: "I need to dial in my obliques and ensure that I have greater separation and size on my quads." Sometimes, daily diet considerations have major health objectives: "I've just been diagnosed with a stage II hepatocellular carcinoma and I want to do everything I can nutritionally to make sure I beat this."

I help my patients zero in on their nutritional health outcomes and then we identify the metabolic state their body needs to be in to support their goals, primarily by controlling insulin across a spectrum of response to appropriate foods. Next, we can begin to model what the distribution of daily caloric density and macronutrients (fats, protein, carbs, and fibers) should look like, helping induce and sustain the metabolic state required for the patient's health goals. Last, we can make choices about which foods will appropriately meet the demands of total daily calories and macronutrient ratios.

Using this approach, every nutritional program becomes a working collaboration between doctor and patient, customized to patient needs and preferences and adaptable to new conditions and requirements over time.

ENHANCE YOUR FOOD PLAN WITH VITAMIN D SUPPLEMENTS

It's a fact that people don't obtain sufficient vitamin D unless they're taking supplements. This is especially true if they live in cold climates with lots of overcast days or have darker skin. But it's also the case for those in sunny, warm areas. Most people wisely limit their sun exposure, knowing that it can cause harm. Our bodies make vitamin D between the skin, kidneys, and liver in response to sunlight exposure. Though it's called a vitamin, it's actually a hormone made from cholesterol (the -*ster*- indicates it's a *ster*oid). It's crucial for bone health as we age and has a range of other benefits. Recently, some studies have suggested that low vitamin D3 increases the risk of hospitalization from COVID-19,[5] but regardless of whether this is related to higher levels typically seen in healthier individuals who spend more time outdoors and perhaps exercising, we do know that there are a myriad of benefits to maintaining higher levels of vitamin D3, from lower susceptibility to infection and colon cancer to frailty in old age. Consider taking a vitamin D3 supplement of 10,000 IU daily.

These patient-focused nutritional programs often end up being representative of vegan/vegetarian, high protein/low carb, Paleo, keto or carnivore, Mediterranean, flexible, intermittent, or elimination diets. But the primary function of a custom-planned nutritional program is to accelerate patients toward their health goals.

A patient with extant CAD evidenced by soft and/or fibrous plaque (and therefore treatable) will benefit from a diet low in saturated fats, those that tend to promote the formation of LDL cholesterol as well as inflammation. The Mediterranean diet—which is one of the best studied diets and which contains little saturated fat, substantial omega-3 fats, and plenty of antioxidants and fiber to help reduce LDL cholesterol and inflammation—would be an ideal starting point in establishing a diet that works for this patient. For patients without CAD, but with metabolic syndrome, type 2 diabetes, and insulin insensitivity, adopting a ketogenic (mostly fat) diet and/or intermittent fasting (not eating within a certain window that is typically longer than normal) is often a good place to start.

To achieve these goals, planning helps enormously. When you know which times you're going to eat and have your meals ready to go in advance, your opportunity for success skyrockets dramatically. Granted, meal planning isn't part of most people's daily routine, and that's okay, as any number of meal prep services can introduce a measure of convenience when it comes to organizing a planned meal program.

HBA1C TEST REFLECTS SUGAR'S DISPOSITION IN YOUR BODY

To establish a quick and sufficiently accurate metric of where you stand on the spectrum of metabolic function, visit a Rite-Aid, Walgreens, or CVS (or simply fire up your Amazon app) and score an HbA1C monitor. One tiny finger prick later, you will have a very useful measure of your metabolic health. HbA1C measures glycation of hemoglobin (how sugared your red blood cells are) and is a good method to understand how metabolism is functioning, over about a ninety-day window. Anything above a 5.6 percent may inspire you to have your levels determined for metrics like fasting insulin, fasted glucose (blood sugar), ghrelin/leptin, testosterone/estradiol, IGF-1, and TSH; more accurately monitor your carbohydrate intake; and perhaps include supplements such as berberine and metformin as part of your daily regimen.

I'm not suggesting that diet is irrelevant, but rather that dietary regimens should be taken with a grain of salt and that other factors not usually included, such as dental hygiene, should be considered.

THE IMPORTANCE OF NUTRITION AND ORAL HEALTH

As you think about how sugar impacts your body and nutritional needs, I also want you to consider your oral health and its connection to the food (nutrition) you put into your mouth. There is a direct connection between nutrition, oral health, longevity, and how they work together.

In recent years, a number of studies have demonstrated that good oral hygiene can improve healthspan and longevity. Studies are providing a growing body of evidence that oral bacteria can travel to the heart and cause inflammation. We're learning that it's not just bad cholesterol that causes heart disease, but also bacteria or viruses that catalyze the inflammatory process in combination with LDL cholesterol. That's why people who are in great shape—they exercise regularly, eat properly, don't smoke, and have excellent lipid panels—can still have arterial blockages.

In his book *If Your Mouth Could Talk,* which won the #1 Medical Nationally Bestselling Book award, Dr. Kami Hoss[6] discusses how good dental care and oral health can keep the body's cardiac and respiratory diseases at bay.

Of course, we know that we should take time to brush and floss our teeth. Dr. Hoss's research outlines how important getting food and its residual bacteria out of our mouth is when it comes to keeping our body healthy. From a healthspan perspective, mouth bacteria accumulate and seep into the body gradually, which can lead to an infection called endocarditis in the inner lining of your heart valves or chambers if mouth bacteria spread into the bloodstream and get attached to your heart. Dr. Hoss also examines the research connecting clogged arteries, inflammation, and infections due to oral bacteria. He further points out that specific oral bacteria can be pulled into your lungs to produce respiratory disease. This sounds scary, and people don't even know that oral health can impact respiratory health. Periodontal disease also gives rise to strokes, heart disease, and diabetes. Years ago, I had a tooth infection that I'm convinced led to a sudden appearance of arterial plaque. I investigated other possible causes, but ultimately, the only logical culprit was the tooth infection.

I believe that in the future, we'll see a much greater emphasis on brushing teeth and flossing, not just to avoid cavities but also to prevent inflammation that can create heart issues. The takeaway here is that regardless of which nutrition protocol you follow, you should visit your dentist for regular checkups and address dental issues as early as possible.

4

Cheating Cancer with Polyphenols

WHEN IT COMES to cheating Death, acknowledging cancer—and the real possibility that it will come for you—is a must. Historically, when cancer showed up, a person's longevity game got much tougher to play; for some it became unwinnable. Death and cancer could be considered teammates.

According to cancer.gov, the leading cause of death *worldwide* is cancer[7]—though, in the United States, heart disease is the leading cause of death, with cancer an extremely close second. In 2018, 18.1 million new cases and 9.5 million cancer-related deaths were reported worldwide. By 2040, 29.5 million new cases and 16.4 million cancer-related deaths are predicted.

Coming from a guy who has always lived a healthy lifestyle and still had to survive both skin and prostate cancer, going head to head with this opponent is anything but easy. The cancer-fighting methods that come to most people's minds are surgery, chemotherapy, radiation, and, more recently, immunotherapy. These are effective oncology tools, and I'm in no way suggesting that people should ignore them in favor of alternatives.

At the same time, we're seeing the further emergence of a wide range of preventive and healing therapies that offer great hope and may even help many cancer patients get the upper hand on Death, now and especially in the future. Alternatives, complements, and adjuncts to cancer therapies that fall outside surgery, chemotherapy, and radiation represent a huge field, and my purpose here isn't to cover all of the products and procedures available. Instead, I want to focus on the ones that I'm most excited about and explain how and why they work.

NOT ALL POLYPHENOLS ARE CREATED EQUAL

The best place to begin is with a discussion of what polyphenols are and why they're beneficial.

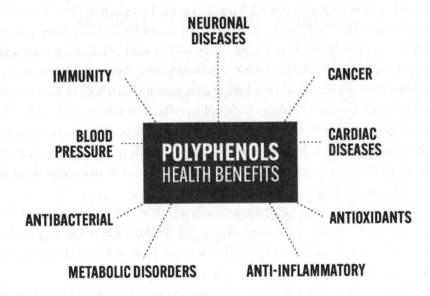

A *polyphenol* is a class of organic compounds similar to alcohols, a bunch of which form a polyphenol. They occur naturally in plants, and one, vanillin, is the main flavoring in vanilla. Other common natural sources are broccoli and tea (from the tannins). Some polyphenols confer health, such as resveratrol found in red wine, epigallocatechin-3-gallate (EGCG) extracted from green tea, and the fraction of curcumin contained in turmeric.

Flavonoids are subclasses of one type of polyphenol that in turn have their own subclasses—flavonols, isoflavones, and others. The polyphenol in green tea and curcumin in turmeric, for instance, are flavonoids. Red wine's resveratrol, on the other hand, is a non-flavonoid polyphenol.

Try this experiment: type "Polyphenols, cancer" into Google. You'll receive almost eight million results. If you narrow your search to "green tea extract, cancer," you'll receive more than thirty-three million hits. About 174,000 of those are peer-reviewed or scholarly articles testifying to its effectiveness. One of the first results is from the Memorial Sloan Kettering Cancer Center website, which recognizes that green tea extract has proven to be a promising anticancer treatment.

Now, let's dig down into how polyphenols work to fight cancer. My friend, colleague, and former college professor, Dr. Gagik Melikyan, deserves credit for first explaining to me the process by which polyphenols function. What he pointed out then and what has stuck with me since is that polyphenols convert to ortho quinones and, as such, can do both harm and good through their effect on cellular DNA. This is especially true of polyphenols that contain ortho-hydroxy groups, such as catechins found in green tea—they oxidize easily, facilitating their ability to destroy cancer cells. It's a similar process to traditional chemotherapy. For instance, daunorubicin is a chemotherapy drug produced naturally by bacteria and used to treat leukemia. Like drugs such as doxorubicin, idarubicin, and epirubicin, daunorubicin is a highly effective anticancer drug that depends on ortho quinones like those in green tea. In addition, anticancer research is focusing a significant amount of effort studying quinones and certain derivatives in an attempt to create effective synthetic preparations.

Other naturally occurring quinones such as juglone (from henna) and emodin (from rhubarb) also have anticancer activity, but the downside is that they exhibit toxicity and attack healthy cells. This has been an issue with traditional chemotherapy as well.

Therefore, the key is to find the sweet spot between toxicity and effectiveness. Polyphenols such as EGCG are less powerful than other ortho quinone methide–derivative drugs for cancer such as anthracyclines, so they're less toxic and safer.

As such, they are useful as preventive measures for early-stage cancers. Because of this less powerful chemotherapeutic trait, many polyphenols are essentially "chemotherapy lite." Admittedly, the studies that demonstrate the viability of polyphenols for this purpose are epidemiological rather than more thorough, rigorous studies. Still, epidemiological studies backed by laboratory investigation suggest the effectiveness of polyphenols in prevention, and, arguably, even treatment of early-stage cancer given what we know about the mechanisms by which polyphenols work.

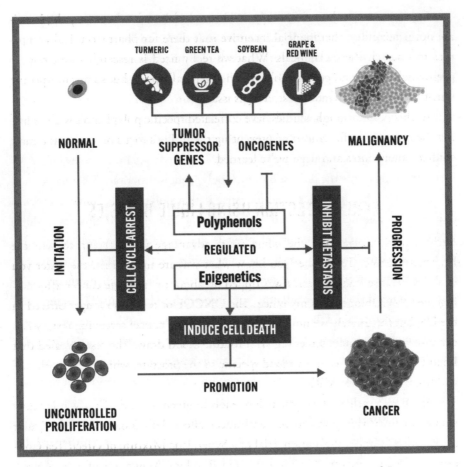

Select Polyphenols and Their Effect on Prevention and Progression of Cancer

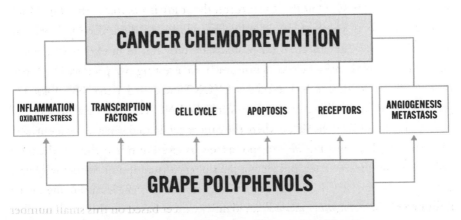

Specific Mechanisms by Which Grape Polyphenols Affect Cancer

Ideally, more studies of this type will be undertaken, but because polyphenols are not proprietary, the financial incentive isn't there for pharmaceutical companies to research these chemicals. What we really need is research about how to improve absorption of polyphenols, which is generally poor, but some enterprising scientists may be motivated to study this issue.

At this point, though, studies have correlated specific polyphenols with reducing the risk of specific cancers or preventing them. Let's focus on one of the most studied polyphenols and what we've learned.

EARLY DETECTION USING LIQUID BIOPSIES

Early detection gives you the home court advantage when trying to win the healthspan game. The sooner you know what you are up against, the faster you can play defense that matters. I was tipped off about my prostate cancer after taking the ONCOblot test in my office. The ONCOblot test is no longer offered in the US, but fortunately we now have GRAIL's Galleri cancer screening test, which can also provide cancer screening via a routine blood draw. The test revealed that I had ENOX2 proteins in my blood specific to the prostate, which was confirmed with multiparametric MRI.

As I noted earlier, one of the polyphenols in green tea is EGCG. While many studies identify this polyphenol's anticancer effect, let's look at one particular study, titled "Cancer Prevention Trial of a Synergistic Mixture of Green Tea Concentrate Plus Capsicum (CAPSOL-T) in a Random Population of 110 Subjects Ages 40–84." This study was conducted by Claudia Hanau, Dr. James Morré, and Dr. Morré's wife, Dorothy. One reason the study is notable is that Dr. Morré spent almost forty years—essentially his life's work—studying ENOX2 proteins and their presence in cancer. These proteins are only found in two places, cancer and fetal development, which is significant from a testing perspective. Dr. Morré developed a test to detect the presence of ENOX2 and called it an ONCOblot Tissue of Origin Cancer Test. In fact, by testing the ENOX2's molecular weight and isoelectric point (pH), the tissue where the cancer originated can also be identified. The test is highly sensitive, able to spot as few as eight hundred thousand cancer cells. That sounds like a lot, but from a physiological standpoint, it's actually very few, typically representing all the cancer cells across a lesion of less than one square millimeter in size. *No other method* can identify cancer based on this small number of cells.

Whether subscribing to the somatic (genetic, in the nucleus of the cell) theory or metabolic (mitochondrial, in the cytoplasm of the cell) theory of cancer development, all agree that cancer forms when mutating cells begin to grow rapidly and out of control. Cell mutations occur in our bodies all the time, but they don't all become cancers because we have a natural process that destroys these mutations. But when this process fails, cancer starts. In these instances, we still possess the capacity to control and even reverse cancer, but we need to intervene early, and "chemotherapy lite" can be a highly effective intervention, as Dr. Morré's study demonstrates.

This study also reveals that it takes more than a cup of green tea daily to control or reverse cancer. The amount of green tea concentrate used in the study was the equivalent of sixteen cups of green tea (concentrated and encapsulated without the energizing constituents such as theophylline and other alkaloids) per serving. The green tea was combined with concentrated capsaicin to facilitate the polyphenol's availability to cells, dramatically increasing its cancer-killing power. When the treated patients were retested for ENOX2 proteins, results showed they were absent, indicating how effective the treatment was.

Along with using it on myself, I've used the ONCOblot test in my practice to identify a number of patients with ENOX2 in their blood. We followed up with additional testing, such as a multiparametric MRI for prostate cancer or mammography and biopsy for breast cancer. Patients who tested positive, including me, underwent 90 to 180 days of treatment with CAPSOL-T (green tea extract with capsaicin). Some of us also combined CAPSOL-T with doses of metformin, depending on the type of cancer and patient circumstances; some also had surgery. Every patient (including myself) tested negative (using ONCOblot) for ENOX2 proteins after these nonsurgical treatments and additional, traditional testing confirmed that the cancer was gone.

HOW TO USE POLYPHENOLS: CAUTIONS AND CONSIDERATIONS

As positive as I am about polyphenols, I also know that even seemingly "harmless" products such as over-the-counter medicines come with a warning. With polyphenols, the warning has to do with toxicity. Too much of anything can be a bad thing, and liver toxicity is a concern with polyphenols if you take too much or are fasting. Perhaps more significantly, they also can have overall systemic and cellular toxicity when used as "chemotherapy lite." Like traditional chemotherapy, polyphenol treatments disrupt DNA beneficially in cancer cells, but also harmfully (though to a much lesser extent than chemo) in healthy cells. Chemo's goal is to target cancer cells while sparing, though wounding, healthy cells. Thus, the polyphenol dose needs to be calibrated judiciously. Ideally, the cancer is caught in the early stages, meaning that the dose doesn't have to be extremely high. If a person you know has ever gone through chemotherapy, they will often say something like, "Yes, the chemo worked to kill the cancer, but it almost killed me first." Too high a dose of polyphenols, like too high a dose of traditional chemo, can devastate healthy cells while destroying cancer cells.

Second, not all polyphenols are created equal. Put another way, one polyphenol may be better for a particular type of cancer than another. In addition, one polyphenol may work particularly well with another polyphenol, or you may want to avoid a particular combination because of potential toxicity or one canceling out the effects of another. For instance, one study suggests that the use of EGCG with curcumin may decrease the efficacy of either cancer-fighting polyphenol.

Third, as I noted earlier, absorption can be a problem with polyphenols. Fortunately, we can improve their bioavailability by combining them with an alkaloid extract of the black pepper family (*Piper nigrum*). We can also combine polyphenols with phospholipids to facilitate absorption.

Fourth, the good news is that polyphenols aren't expensive and don't require prescriptions. They do require consultation with a doctor who has experience using them to treat particular types of cancer in order to figure out the right ones to use as well as the doses. From a preventive medicine standpoint, however, everyone can take advantage of their cancer-fighting properties. Empirically, there's evidence to suggest that because the French drink so much red wine and the Japanese so much green tea in combination with other polyphenols from other sources as well as other positive lifestyle routines, they have better health and longevity than many other populations.

WHY POLYPHENOLS (AND OTHER ALTERNATIVE APPROACHES) AREN'T THE STANDARD OF CARE

None of my enthusiasm for polyphenols makes me ignore the continued need for surgery, chemo, radiation, and immunotherapy, especially for advanced forms of cancer. All the same, I'm also aware that the business of medicine causes doctors to be less aware of and enthusiastic about polyphenols than they should be.

Long before I became a doctor, I read an article about Dr. Bjorn Nordenstrom, a Swedish physician who experimented by inserting cathodes into tumors. This treatment was successful, presumably by attracting negatively charged white blood cells to the tumor and killing them. The article's author asked prominent doctors if they were aware of Nordenstrom's work and why doctors in the US weren't practicing and researching similar treatments. While these doctors admitted that Nordenstrom's work was impressive, they explained that they were focused on their own methods for treating cancer—methods that had much greater potential for research funding.

Similarly, there isn't as much financial incentive for scientists to research anti-cancer treatments using polyphenols as there is for other, more lucrative approaches. We're also now seeing greater medical-community recognition of alternative methods and the value of naturally occurring chemicals like polyphenols. As someone who began his career studying nutrition, moved on to naturopathic and orthomolecular medicine, studied traditional Chinese medicine, and then went to medical school, I've witnessed a shift in attitude and practice regarding alternative and complementary methods.

POLYPHENOLS' HISTORY OF USE

Traditional Chinese medicine as well as Indian Ayurvedic medicine use herbs and herbal formulations containing polyphenols to fight cancer.

Admittedly—and unfortunately—it's difficult to create credibility for forms of medicine such as acupuncture, where you can't do the double-blinded, placebo-controlled studies that provide scientific validity. Polyphenols, however, are chemicals that can and should be studied more using rigorous scientific methods.

It's time we become even more open-minded about how we treat the illnesses and disorders that confront us, whether they are viruses, aging-related issues, or cancer.

5

Cheating Death with
Dietary Supplements

AN ESTIMATED 77 percent of Americans take dietary supplements including herbs, vitamins, amino acids, enzymes, minerals, and other substances.[8] Yet one problem with supplements is that a lot of misinformation exists about which ones people should take. One year there's a study that advocates a particular vitamin or mineral, the next year there's a new study that cautions people against it. In addition, advertising claims may exaggerate benefits and not jibe with actual research results. Confusion reigns and the internet lights up with all sorts of uninformed perspectives.

Another problem is that things change quickly. We're learning a lot more about the value of supplements every day, but this information takes a while to reach everyone and gain acceptance. So, while my purpose here isn't to give you a laundry list of supplements, I want to focus on the particular ones that have the most significant effect on healthspan and raise awareness of specific types that aren't as well known as they should be.

A CAUTION ABOUT REGENERATIVE SUPPLEMENTS

If you read the label on just about any supplement bottle today, you will see convincing language that you should be taking said supplement for a myriad of positive health benefits. While vitamins and various nutrients categorized as supplements definitely can optimize health, two caveats are worth mentioning.

Many of you may recall hearing about the "amazing" benefits of vitamin B12 in promoting energy, even "weight (fat) loss." People often swear by its ability to perk them up under almost any circumstance, and a major weight-loss company claims that large doses of vitamin B12 can help people lose fat. Many of you also may have tried vitamin B12 and thought it was underwhelming in effect, left wondering either what is so special about it or whether something was wrong with you. Like a car that has plenty of oil, for which adding another quart won't make a difference in the way the car runs, so, too, are you just carrying around an extra quart of B12 "oil" after such large doses on top of an adequate supply. However, if your car is running very low or out of oil, engine performance will improve dramatically when you replenish the oil.

One of the issues with supplements is that, while there are regulations in place for their manufacture, sourcing, and use, as well as about claims made regarding their function and efficacy, there is woefully little enforcement of these regulations. Finding a supplement of quality can be an issue. Too many times, a supplement has been written off as ineffective when the supplement used was not of sufficient quality or quantity as advertised on the label. You should buy supplements provided by manufacturers who use third-party independent testing to provide assays confirming the content and purity of their products. A list of some supplement manufacturers I recommend and trust:

- Designs for Health
- Jarrow
- Life Extension Foundation
- Thorne
- Pure Encapsulations
- Integrative Therapeutics

Be judicious in your selection of supplements by testing for nutrients in blood assays—essentially, find out if your figurative oil is a quart low. In addition, keep one of my favorite traditional Chinese medicine terms in mind as you survey supplements. Chinese medicine practitioners talk about "superior herbs" as describing certain supplements that are not taken to treat an ailment or deficiency but rather to improve brain function, reduce inflammation, strengthen the immune system, and provide other health advantages. If you are intent on optimizing health and have not identified any particular issues with your current state, the following supplements are good starting points.

Now, let's get into the longevity supplements I think are worth pointing out, getting to know, and adding to your healthspan tool box—these are real ways to cheat Death!

A BEST-KEPT LONGEVITY SECRET: NAD+

If you ask people, "What's a good supplement?" they're likely to answer with vitamin C or calcium. Nothing is wrong with these answers, but they're unlikely to name one substance especially important for anyone concerned about their healthspan: NAD+. Let's look at why this would have been an excellent response.

Nicotinamide adenine dinucleotide (NAD+) is a coenzyme, or molecule that is crucial for cell functioning and energy metabolism; the plus at the end just means that it's missing an electron. There are actually two forms of NAD in our body, NAD+ and NADH; the latter is converted from NAD+ and both are necessary for our mitochondria to function effectively, turning food and oxygen into energy. Though there's some debate among scientists about the ratio of NAD+ to NADH versus the amount of NAD+ in our bodies, we know that the ratio is important because it determines how well cells can produce ATP, our cells' primary source of energy.

IMPROVING CELL FUNCTION WITH NAD+

NAD+ also activates so-called sirtuin proteins essential for regulating cellular health and helps modify proteins for cell signaling, which improves cellular function.

We produce some of the NAD+ we need naturally by eating food with NAD+ precursors—everything from dairy to fish to mushrooms. These foods contain the vitamin B3, the base for NAD+. Combining these foods with tryptophan (found in turkey and other foods) helps produce NAD+. We can't make sufficient NAD+ from our diet, so our bodies recycle leftover nicotinamide (after the NAD+ has fulfilled its cell-signaling function) using what is referred to as the "salvage pathway." Notably, we produce the lion's share of our NAD+ as a result of exercising, adding yet another benefit to regular exercise.

The big issue is whether supplements can help NAD+ reach deep into the cell where it does the most good and into all cells of the body, as opposed to when ingested as a supplement, following which it collects and remains in the liver.

My experience, both from my patients who have taken NAD+ supplements and from a review of the research, is that these supplements have multiple beneficial effects for all the reasons previously listed, even if there's some debate over how the biological mechanism functions. We know that as we age, we lose NAD+. We also know that NAD+ plays a major role in DNA maintenance and repair and that, without sufficient NAD+, this function starts to break down. In addition, NAD+ is protective against cancer because of its cell repair role and scientists are exploring various ways to incorporate NAD+ into different cancer therapies.

Research is currently being conducted using NAD+ to develop new antibiotics. Because some antibiotics have been overprescribed and are no longer as effective as they once were, novel antibiotics are needed. NAD+ offers a fresh way to do so through its mechanism of action in mammals.

In addition, studies are underway exploring NAD+'s effectiveness in treating Parkinson's disease, Alzheimer's disease, and other neurodegenerative illnesses. For instance, they've found that nicotinamide riboside (NR), a supplemental source for the production of NAD+, may have neuroprotective effects, shielding brain cells from the damage caused by Alzheimer's.

To call NAD+ a miracle supplement is an overstatement, but it does have a remarkably wide range of benefits. We can generate more NAD+ in a variety of ways: exercise, fasting, and consuming (e.g., resveratrol, the plant compound found in red wine, helps activate sirtuin genes) are just some possibilities. Taking a supplement is the easiest path to capitalizing on NAD+'s healthspan benefits, although I would assert that exercise is *better* because of all its additional potential benefits. NR seems to be the best supplement, and the usual dose is up to 1,000 mg daily; the body converts it into NAD+. One of the best effects of this supplement is that it helps create a better ratio between NAD+ and NADH.

While other supplements exist that have a positive NAD+ effect, NR seems like the best one as of this writing. If you're considering it, it's also wise to combine its use with a "methyl donor" such as supplemental choline (500 mg/day), S-adenosyl L-methionine (SAMe; 400–600 mg/day), or natural sources such as eggs (three per day) because NR can consume methyl groups when metabolized.

Another option is intravenous NAD+, which raises levels higher than oral intake since it's better absorbed. The intravenous method also has a greater effect on cell signaling, resetting the cells so they function better. Though a lot more research has to be done, the early indications are that this intravenous approach also produces better sleep by restoring circadian rhythms, lessens depression, and provides more energy. In addition, this approach is being explored as a way to treat addictions.

From a long-term perspective, NAD+ has a positive impact on longevity. By using NAD+ supplements or stimulating our bodies to make more of it through diet or exercise, we increase our genomic stability, because a better NAD+-to-NADH ratio facilitates DNA repair. The analogy used by David Sinclair, Harvard Medical School professor of genetics and longevity expert, bears repeating. The main cause of aging is what he terms "a scratch on the CD" or corruption of the DNA, the crucial information and set of instructions that reside in our cells. NAD+ protects us against developing these flaws and helps repair them while helping lengthen our cells' telomeres.[9]

SENOLYTICS

This term refers to drugs, supplements, and chemicals that target cells that have reached senescence (i.e., have stopped dividing and are no longer functioning optimally) in order to limit the damage of cancerous or otherwise problematic cells. Our bodies naturally destroy some of these cells, but others linger and accelerate the aging process. Harvard Medical School's David Sinclair talks about how the aging process is a result of corrupted DNA, and how eliminating cells with this corruption could have a positive effect on how we age. Removing senescent cells, though, is tricky—it has to be a highly targeted process.

Studies have been undertaken in which certain senolytic drugs that home in on senescent cells have demonstrated efficacy, including daptomycin and quercetin, fisetin, piperlongumine, *Rosa canina*, *Panax notoginseng*, and curcumin. Many other drugs and supplements are currently being studied, and the hope is that some will prove superior in targeting senescence. This would represent a major step forward for our healthspans, while helping prevent disease and facilitating improved athletic performance.

BOOST IMMUNITY AND TELOMERE LENGTH WITH AC-11

A patented extract of a rainforest plant species found in Brazil and Peru, AC-11 is a water-soluble extract of the inner bark of the supplement sold under the name "cat's claw." It's been found to have many beneficial effects, but two key cellular effects are its ability to decrease DNA damage and to lengthen telomeres. Studies indicate that taking 350 mg of AC-11 daily yields significant telomere lengthening after 12 months and even more lengthening after 24 months. Though you'll probably be tired of this analogy by the end of the book, it's apt: DNA damage is like a scratch on a CD, hurting its quality at best and rendering it inoperable at worst. Being able to repair the damage done and reduce future damage can be major pluses for healthspan.

AC-11 also supports healthy immune function. An overactive immune system produces allergies and other problems, while an underactive one can allow cancer cells to flourish. AC-11 facilitates a balanced immune system. This is especially important as we age, since our immune function tends to become dysregulated and upregulated. As a result, we suffer from a variety of ills—arthritis and gastritis as well as pancreatic and colon cancer. In its role as a cell regulator, AC-11 helps mitigate the effects of aging on our immune system. For instance, apoptosis is the natural ability of our bodies to kill cells, one that is essential as we attempt to fight off cancer—apoptosis kills cancer cells, too. As we age, however, this ability diminishes; AC-11 may be able to restore it.

In addition, some studies (human as well as animal) indicate that AC-11 can reverse skin damage caused by the sun's UV rays. I've also used AC-11 to enhance the effectiveness of stem cell treatments by treating the patient with AC-11 to optimize the cells before harvesting them.

Again, all these benefits make it seem like AC-11 supplements should be widely embraced by the healthcare establishment and sold by Big Pharma, but this isn't the case. Part of the problem is that there isn't a lot of money to be made from obtaining the cat's claw plant used to make AC-11 from the rainforest. A company has obtained the rights to sell a patented cat's claw extract, but it isn't making a lot of money doing so.

Given the relatively few potential serious side effects and cautions, however (including dizziness and nausea associated with cat's claw, but not with AC-11), AC-11 is definitely a promising supplement worth considering to enhance healthspan.

IMPROVE BLOOD FLOW AND PERFORMANCE WITH L-CARNOSINE

L-carnosine is a supplement popular with people (especially athletes) who want to delay the effects of aging on the body. L-carnosine acts as a pH buffer for the cells and has the ability to agonize (activate) endothelial nitric oxide synthase, increasing production of nitric oxide, which opens up blood vessels. As a result, it creates better blood flow to various key areas of the body—the heart, brain, and sex organs. L-carnosine provides athletes with such a significant benefit that it should probably be considered an unfair advantage.

L-carnosine is difficult to absorb via the gastrointestinal tract, so the best source for oral supplementation is through beta-alanine, a combination of L-carnosine and L-histidine that is easily absorbed. Athletes take it (most effectively in a sustained-release form of beta-alanine) because it may boost their workout performance; they may obtain greater endurance and ability to engage in high-intensity exercise because of L-carnosine's ability to buffer the buildup of acid in the cell, which results from anaerobic energy production. I recommend taking 2 to 4 grams by mouth per day of a sustained-release form of beta-alanine.

THE DIFFERENCE BETWEEN L-CARNOSINE AND L-CARNITINE

L-carnosine should not be confused with another supplement and ergogenic aid, L-carnitine. L-carnitine can be used by athletes and others who want to leverage the use of fat for energy, and studies show its use can increase time-to-exhaustion by 20 percent. L-carnitine is not a regenerative tool, but it certainly deserves mention as an ergogenic supplement (20 percent more time to exhaustion could provide a significant boost in performance, helping the user secure the top spot on the podium or even just making the team!). It can also help keep fat off and teach the body to use fat as fuel over muscle glycogen.

PROTECT GOOD ESTROGEN WITH INDOLE-3-CARBINOL

Indole-3-carbinol (IC3) is composed of substances found in cruciferous vegetables (cauliflower, broccoli, cabbage, etc.). IC3 protects us from a negative estrogen-conversion process as we age (for both men and women—*men also produce estrogen*). When we pass the age when we can reproduce, our bodies stop converting bad estrogens into neutral or good estrogens. A urinary 2/16 alpha hydroxye-strone test can determine if our ratio of good (2-hydroxyestrone) to bad estro-gen (16-alpha-hydroxyestrone) has moved in the wrong direction, which makes women more vulnerable to breast cancer and men to prostate cancer. To prevent this negative trend, we can eat a lot of cruciferous vegetables. We can also take IC3 (or another close metabolite, diindolylmethane, or DIM), which has been shown to promote the conversion of bad estrogen (4-hydroxyestrone is also considered a harmful estrogen) to good. I recommend taking 100 to 200 mg orally of DIM per day with food.

PROMOTE OPTIMAL CELLULAR FUNCTION AND REDUCE TENSION WITH MAGNESIUM

Magnesium is probably the best-known supplement I'll mention in this section. Magnesium treatment improved mitochondrial ATP synthesis and greater ATP availability as a result, which is necessary for cellular energy supply and survival. Magnesium treatment also consistently improved longevity in mice and reduced their vascular calcification. Most of us have probably forgotten our high school physiology, but in order to convert food into usable cellular energy, the Krebs cycle (a.k.a. the citric acid cycle) requires many nutrients including Coenzyme Q10, zinc, manganese, most of the B-vitamins, and . . . *magnesium!* Without it, our cells do not function optimally and our health suffers.

Most adults have low levels of or are actually deficient in magnesium. While it naturally occurs in common foods—salmon, spinach, bran cereals, almonds—many people don't get enough. When we're under a lot of stress, we burn through our magnesium, and many of us are under significant stress these days. Magne-sium provides a number of beneficial functions. It facilitates blood flow, assists in the production of energy, and helps us relax (and get a good night's sleep). Studies show type A people especially experience a beneficial blood pressure reduction when taking magnesium supplements.

Magnesium is generally poorly absorbed (which is why it can function as a good laxative; think "milk of magnesia"), but three supplements that stand out are: mag-nesium glycinate (since it is comparatively well absorbed), magnesium threonate (which can cross the blood–brain barrier better than the others), or magnesium tau-rate (which offers more in terms of calming effects). The best way to measure mag-nesium is from cells—specifically red blood cells—rather than via blood serum.

SQUELCH INFLAMMATION WITH CURCUMIN

Curcumin is another supplement that might be familiar to you in that it's a derivative of the spice turmeric. Consuming a gram of curcumin twice daily helps reduce inflammation. In fact, in my practice, I've seen patients who—after taking curcumin for three weeks—have the same amount of pain reduction as they would taking NSAIDs. NSAIDs have been linked to kidney and gastrointestinal issues; their use now is considered the number-one cause of stomach ulcers. And, for those with gout and elevated uric acid levels, curcumin is an excellent first choice to evaluate for its effectiveness in resolving symptoms of inflammation and pain while reducing uric acid levels.

Note that, while turmeric contains the active constituent curcumin, taking turmeric will not have the same effect as taking curcumin. By the time the body can extract the curcumin from turmeric, it is well down the digestive tract and turmeric use will likely only benefit inflammation of the colon. Curcumin extracts that use nanoparticle technology or piperine derivatives to enhance absorbability should be taken rather than turmeric. Curcumin also seems to help prevent pancreatic cancer in some people. I'm not suggesting that curcumin is better than NSAIDs for all conditions or all individuals, but it is an option worth considering for reducing inflammation, especially if one has been chronically using NSAIDs.[10]

FIGHT HEALTH INVADERS WITH GLUTATHIONE + VITAMIN C

The combination of vitamin C and glutathione is a good way to fight fungus, viruses, and bacterial infections. Glutathione is a natural antioxidant in the body, though we produce it less and less as we age, and vitamin C, an antioxidant in its own right, helps supercharge it. Because glutathione is difficult to absorb, taking the supplement N-acetyl-cysteine instead remedies the absorbability problem associated with glutathione through the digestive tract, converting to glutathione in the liver and enabling vitamin C to function more effectively as an antioxidant.

OTHER ITEMS TO CONSIDER IN YOUR "CHEATING DEATH" SUPPLEMENT CABINET

I'm not going to spend a lot of time discussing some of the most well-known supplements—omega-3 fatty acids, B complex, and vitamin D3—but they're all excellent for most people. Two grams of fish oil (which contains omega-3s) daily is usually the minimum dose to reduce inflammation and keep blood platelets from sticking together. A capsule of most typical B-complex vitamins with each meal is probably a bare minimum to keep up with most individuals' level of stress, and 5,000 to 10,000 IU of vitamin D3 per day (also taken with food) should optimize levels of these substances. There are several other supplements worth considering that may or may not provide sufficient "juice for the squeeze" such as astaxanthin, apigenin, sulforaphane, astragalus, melatonin, and pyridoxamine. As always, a visit with one's regenerative medicine physician would be helpful in sussing out the value of these and other substances in each individual circumstance.

CONDITIONS THAT CAN BE HELPED WITH SUPPLEMENTATION

Here are a few specific conditions for which I've found other types of supplements to be effective:

Non-Alcoholic Fatty Liver Disease: According to the American Liver Foundation, the number of Americans with non-alcoholic fatty liver disease (NAFLD) is estimated at 100 million. That's a lot of people whose livers contain excess fat, a problem that produces fatigue, abdominal pain, low energy, and can also lead to cirrhosis, a potentially fatal disease. Even though it can be asymptomatic for long stretches, NAFLD's long-term effects can harm one's healthspan.

NAFLD is a modern occurrence, a result of our industrialized culture in which people combine overeating with a lack of exercise. After we use energy stored as glycogen in a muscle, food eaten is used to refuel the muscle's glycogen stores. But once that glycogen is replenished, its next stop for any excess blood sugar is the liver, where it is stored as fat.

To prevent or remedy fatty liver disease, we often need to avoid oversupplying the depleted muscle with excess energy. Here's a simple suggestion: balance energy-expending outputs such as daily exercise with energy inputs such as calorie-rich food and drink. A corollary to this oversimplification is to avoid eating foods with a high glycemic index (an index of individually consumed foods that measures how quickly and highly the blood sugar climbs in the blood) or too much food at once (overwhelming the body's ability to balance calories consumed with those used so that the "excess at the moment" is stored as fat). A less simple but effective alternative is frequently recommended for people with a genetic predisposition to or extant fatty liver: supplementing with a combination of the amino acid L-methionine, choline (the methyl donor and B vitamin referenced earlier), and inositol (also a B vitamin). This approach can typically reverse fatty liver in as little as thirty days. No pharmaceutical treatment currently available for NAFLD can work this effectively and quickly. Methyl donors are especially important for treatment of fatty liver disease because some people are genetically predisposed to struggle with the condition.

Bodybuilders have long been aware of the curative value of this combination of supplements for NAFLD. In fact, I first learned of the use of choline and inositol to treat fatty liver from Dr. Franco Columbu, the famous bodybuilder and multiple-time Mr. Olympia. Some bodybuilders would use anabolic steroids to facilitate deposition of as much energy as possible in muscles. They would then overeat and not move much in an effort to "bulk up," knowing they would often develop fatty livers, for which they could count on the combination of choline and inositol (we have since added L-methionine, too) to resolve. To be clear, lifting weights isn't correlated with NAFLD, but taking anabolic steroids, having poor nutrition, and not getting enough exercise can lead to NAFLD. Bodybuilders simply began taking these supplements to counteract the effect of their regimens because they found them to be effective.

The recommended dosages to counter NAFLD are:

- 1,500 mg of methionine
- 3,000 mg of choline
- 3,000 mg of inositol

As noted, usually after thirty days, fatty liver disease resolves. Every so often, a patient comes in with a case of fatty liver diagnosed by their primary care physician and confirmed with imaging such as abdominal ultrasound. They're understandably concerned, especially because their doctors had no easy remedy. I'm always happy to provide the remedy of a thirty-day course of daily "MIC caps" (L-methionine, inositol, choline) in the doses just described. Most physicians can't believe something so simple and easy can do the trick, but they are, of course, happy to see the results and then adopt the remedy for other patients.

An effort is now underway to get these three ingredients classified as a medical food, which would allow doctors to write prescriptions for them, making it more likely that insurance would provide reimbursement. But even without reimbursement, a thirty-day supply of these supplements is relatively affordable at approximately $200 for a 30-day supply. For those who tend to be prone to fatty liver, I recommend either a daily prophylactic dose equal to half of the thirty-day treatment dose or periodic "treatment" before too much fat accumulates in the liver.

Sleep Issues: Serotonin precursors include such compounds as 5-hydroxytryptophan (5-HTP) or L-tryptophan. Serotonin is a hormone and a neurotransmitter that affects our moods, providing us with a sense of well-being; for me, it's that feeling as a kid when I woke up on a weekend morning and smelled the pancakes and bacon cooking. Many antidepressants are selective serotonin reuptake inhibitors (SSRIs) that increase brain levels of serotonin, which helps relax us. By taking 5-HTP or L-tryptophan, we are providing the body with more precursors to serotonin, and often— simply based upon the principles of stoichiometry (the relationship between quantities of a compound in a chemical reaction)—the body will make more serotonin, leaving one more relaxed and helping us sleep better. SSRI antidepressants are much stronger in effect, but 5-HTP and L-tryptophan are powerful enough that they should not be taken with SSRIs, because doing so can cause unwanted and even dangerous side effects.

Consider supplementing with:

- 200 mg of 5-HTP 200-1, by mouth, 30 to 60 minutes before bedtime if you are having difficulty sleeping

TURKEY DOESN'T MAKE YOU SLEEPY

Contrary to popular belief—and the fact that 5-HTP is a component of L-tryptophan—the tryptophan in turkey doesn't help us sleep. Turkey has been mistaken for a sleep aid because after a big meal at Thanksgiving, we tend to sleep soundly, but most animal proteins contain significant amounts of L-tryptophan. In reality, it's usually because we overate, and the experience of a postprandial (after-eating) narcosis or "food coma," or overindulging in alcohol, that caused us to feel sleepy.

Muscle Aches Due to Statins: Coenzyme Q10 (CoQ10). A nutrient that occurs naturally in the body, CoQ10 has been found to ease muscle pain in some people who take statins for CAD. When experiencing statin-induced muscle aches—in addition to considering alternative statins or alternatives to statins such as red yeast rice—you may want to add CoQ10 to the regimen.

Consider supplementing with:

- 400–800 mg of CoQ10 per day, as a trial, by mouth

We know that statins leach CoQ10 from cells, and I have found this a worthwhile trial in many patients who experience muscle aches with statin use.

LDL Cholesterol: Red yeast rice. Speaking of statins, not everyone can tolerate their side effects, and some people opt for alternatives such as red yeast rice. It contains at least twenty-five LDL-cholesterol-lowering monacolins including monacolin K, the same ingredient that's in lovastatin; it also helps reduce the formation of low-density lipoproteins (LDL cholesterol, also known and inappropriately referred to as "bad" cholesterol). Red yeast rice can be used to effectively lower LDL cholesterol and typically without many, if any, of the side effects associated with statin drugs.

Consider supplementing with:

- up to 4,800 mg of red yeast rice, by mouth, per day

Arthritis: Methyl donors. Even since drugs such as Vioxx, Celebrex, and other NSAIDs were taken off the market because of concerns about side effects, especially heart problems, people with arthritis pain have not had a lot of effective options to deal with their disease. Methyl donor supplements such as creatine, glycine, choline, and others have been shown to be effective in reducing this type of pain. Also, consider adding curcumin to supplant the use of NSAIDs.

Consider supplementing with:

- 5–15 grams of creatine monohydrate per day
- 3–6 grams of glycine twice per day
- 150 mg of Alpha-GPC twice per day or 250 mg of Cognizin twice per day
- curcumin, 1 gram twice per day

6

Using Sleep to Live
Longer and Better

WE'VE KNOWN THE benefits of getting a good night's rest for years. Here are some of the incentives for obtaining consistently good sleep:

- Helps maintain a healthy weight
- Lowers risk for diabetes and heart problems
- Strengthens the immune system
- Reduces stress
- Lessens risk of depression
- Improves concentration and ability to get work done
- Impacts longevity positively

What's new, though, is the specific knowledge we've gained about how to maximize sleep to benefit our healthspan. Commonly referred to as "the four pillars of sleep," they work together to produce a healthy night's sleep. These pillars are duration (seven to nine hours), depth/quality (based on moving through all the stages of sleep, from light to REM to deep, often dreamless), continuity (sleeping without numerous waking periods), and regularity (going to bed and waking at roughly the same time every day).

Therefore, it's not enough to get eight hours of sleep nightly if you're waking up all the time or if your bedtimes vary.

THE VALUE OF SLEEP FOR HEALTHSPAN

We've learned a lot about sleep, through both research and patients' experiences. I'm going to share this knowledge with you and demonstrate how you can use it to your best advantage.

The benefits of a good night's sleep are multifaceted and significant, but many of us fail to realize these benefits, often because we have misconceptions about sleep. I have patients who arrive in my office, water bottle in hand, having just come from intense workouts at the gym. They exercise vigorously and regularly, get enough water, and eat the right foods. They complain, however, that they can't put any muscle on their bodies.

During our conversations, they admit that they only get four or five hours of sleep nightly. They're working high-stress jobs and either can't sleep a lot because of stress or convince themselves that all they need is a few hours of sleep. What they don't realize is that this lack of sleep is preventing their bodies from operating properly; they're up at night when they should be sleeping, facilitating rest, repairing damage, and translating their earlier workouts into muscle.

Seven to nine hours of sleep is considered optimal. A small percentage of the population has a mutant gene that allows them to function normally and healthfully with less than this amount. But the vast majority of us lack this mutation, even though it's common for people to say things like, "I do fine with four hours of sleep and an occasional nap."

To paraphrase Al Gore, it's an inconvenient truth that we need seven to nine hours of sleep each night. Consider that we're the only animal that deprives its body of sleep for reasons other than starvation or running away from a forest fire in the middle of the night. Our bodies thrive on regularity—our internal clock or, more accurately, our circadian rhythms tell us when to eat, sleep, and wake. When we adhere to these rhythms, our body releases hormones and efficiently performs other processes behind the scenes. When we stick to this schedule, these processes work together synergistically; when we don't, we receive clear signals that something is off. For instance, if you skip lunch, your body, anticipating mealtime, secretes hormones and you feel hunger pangs or hear your stomach growl as a result.

MAJOR HEALTH CHALLENGES CREATED BY POOR SLEEP QUALITY

When we don't get sufficient sleep, we may not receive such immediately recognizable signals; though if we're aware, we probably notice we're sleepier than usual during the day and not always thinking as clearly as we normally do. Inside of us, however, we are incurring harm through a myriad of dysfunctional processes that begin to accumulate, secondary to a lack of sleep.

Insulin Resistance: Dr. Matthew Walker, a professor of psychology and neuroscience at the University of California at Berkeley, is the world's leading expert on sleep. In his book *Why We Sleep: Unlocking the Power of Sleep and Dreams*, Dr. Walker contends that if you go five consecutive days without sufficient sleep, getting only six hours per night—remember, most people require seven to nine hours per night—your insulin sensitivity declines by as much as 50 percent. Reduced insulin sensitivity (or insulin resistance) is associated with heart disease, weight gain, Alzheimer's disease, and cancer.

Weight Gain: Gaining weight is a particularly troubling aspect of not getting sufficient sleep, given the rising obesity rates in the US. As little as a 10 percent drop in insulin sensitivity causes a significant weight gain; just imagine the extra pounds a 50 percent reduction produces. While exercise can counter some of the negative effects of reduced insulin sensitivity—and I'd recommend establishing a good exercise routine if you're not getting enough sleep—a better healthspan strategy is combining exercise with more hours of sleep.

Memory Issues: Problems with memory that don't involve Alzheimer's can also be an issue when you don't sleep well. Research has found that people often struggle with "consolidation"—they fail to integrate what they learned that day during sleep. Lack of sleep also affects mood. When I was a kid, my parents sometimes let me stay up late on a Friday night to watch *Creature Features*. While I still got my eight or nine hours of sleep, I slept much later than usual and often woke up (and stayed) grumpy because I'd shifted my circadian rhythm. Imagine not only shifting your circadian rhythm around every night, but also not getting the requisite amount of good quality sleep *every* night. *Disaster!*

Sexual Dysfunction: Most obviously, if you're tired all the time, you may lack the energy for sex. If you're not fully rested, your sex hormones are also affected. Lack of sleep diminishes levels of luteinizing hormone. Normally, this hormone goes to either the ovaries or testicles, instructing them to produce more testosterone, which affects the libido as well as the production of eggs and sperm.

Autophagy Interruption: This cellular rest-and-repair process enters high gear while we sleep. More specifically, as we switch from the go-go sympathetic (fight or flight) nervous system employed while we're awake to the slow-slow parasympathetic (repair and recover) nervous system that takes over when we sleep, autophagy is more active. Without sufficient rest (read: sleep of both good quality and quantity), the cellular rest and repair processes, including autophagy, cannot be performed. Especially with sleep apnea leading to hypoxia—a medical way of saying you are not getting enough oxygen while you sleep, most often because of snoring—you're going into oxygen debt, just as you might during vigorous exercise. When this happens during sleep, you're preventing these aforementioned processes from operating efficiently or at all. This autophagy problem is particularly acute for our digestive health. The digestive tract is the area of the body where there's the greatest turnover of cells, so if it's not cleaned up regularly—the purpose of autophagy—then we experience digestive issues.

Excess Cortisol: Be aware, too, that without proper sleep, your body produces excess cortisol, the fight-or-flight hormone, to compensate for your lack of energy. While useful in certain situations, chronic cortisol release is terrible for your overall health. Being in a frequent state of wanting to fight or flee has an adverse effect on many areas of the body, stressing us out unnecessarily. If you are under chronic stress and notice that your extremities are lean, but no matter how hard you try, your midsection seems to be retaining fat, chronic cortisol excess is usually a significant part of the problem.

Aging: In addition, aging makes sleep more difficult—it's theorized that our loss of melatonin and/or dysfunction of the pineal gland as we become older makes insomnia more common.

APNEA AND OTHER IMPEDIMENTS TO LIVING LONG, LIVING WELL

The other big obstacle is sleep apnea—the frequent stopping and starting of breathing while we sleep. It can typically take two forms:

- *Obstructive Sleep Apnea,* where the throat muscles relax, the tongue falls back into the airway, the turbinates (filters in the nasal passages) become too large, or a deviated septum blocks one of the sinus passages
- *Central Sleep Apnea,* where the brain fails to send the right signals to the muscles that control breathing

It is possible to suffer from both forms simultaneously. Dr. Walker estimates that 80 percent of people with sleep apnea are undiagnosed. The most common symptom is snoring, but your partner may not even be aware of or concerned about your snoring, or you may be single and not have anyone who alerts you about this symptom.

In my practice, I've found that about 65 percent of my patients have previously undiagnosed sleep apnea. When our patients begin testosterone replacement therapy, blood tests (hemoglobin, hematocrit, and red blood cell count) often reveal this undiagnosed sleep apnea. Physicians as well as lay people often mistake the treatment (testosterone replacement) with the underlying disease (sleep apnea). Testosterone is needed to make red blood cells and hemoglobin, both of which are the body's oxygen-carrying mechanism within the blood. As we age and testosterone decreases, we produce fewer red blood cells and less hemoglobin. Meanwhile, as we age and the soft palate and/or neck muscles become more lax, the tongue grows bigger, the turbinates enlarge, and other causes of sleep apnea manifest as the body's demand for hemoglobin and red blood cells increases. This process is similar to when athletes train beyond their anaerobic threshold and go into "oxygen debt," and in response, the body says, "Well, if you are not going to slow down and/or breathe any faster for oxygen's sake, then we will just have to make more oxygen-carrying capacity (red blood cells and hemoglobin)." The two phenomena oppose each other; therefore, sleep apnea is not typically noted within laboratory assays until testosterone is replaced.

Some of my patients are quick to note the relationship between endurance athletes' desire to increase red blood cell count and hemoglobin suggest that their sleep apnea will allow them to skip regular cardiovascular exercise. While I appreciate their astute observation, two problems exist with their suggestion. First, while red blood cell count and hemoglobin are an essential part of cardiovascular fitness, these are not the entirety of it. Chemical buffering within the muscle cells and mitochondrial development are also essential, and since one is not exercising muscles during apneic sleep, but rather essentially just holding one's breath, overall cardiovascular fitness is not improved with sleep apnea. Second, even if one did receive all the benefits of cardiovascular exercise with sleep apnea, the process is occurring when other essential processes that cannot be displaced are occurring. Autophagy—cellular regeneration and repair—and other essential processes that occur during sleep, along with parasympathetic nervous system activation, won't happen if one is essentially "training in one's sleep" and doing so in what is very often sympathetic nervous system mode; being in oxygen debt and literally gasping for oxygen-containing air.

Ear, nose, and throat doctors suspect sleep apnea when male patients' neck sizes exceed seventeen inches in circumference—thick necks often are accompanied by narrow throat passageways, whether created by muscle or fat deposits, and can obstruct the airway, especially when lying supine.

Being overweight, however, is the main cause of sleep apnea. The apnea makes it difficult to get a good night's sleep, poor sleep produces decreased insulin sensitivity, this sensitivity leads to weight gain, and the weight gain catalyzes sleep apnea. Also, the stress that sleep apnea induces can result in significant hormone imbalances, including reduced thyroid and testosterone production as well as increased cortisol and insulin production. As you can see, this is a vicious cycle, one that you should strive to break by doing whatever your doctor suggests to treat your apnea.

BETTER SLEEP BASICS

Some of these suggestions are widely known, but let's start out by emphasizing certain basics:

- **Don't eat before bedtime.** More specifically, don't consume high-glycemic-load foods and beverages before going to sleep. Ideally, finish your dinner or dessert at least three hours before you get into bed.

This prevents your body temperature from rising; you sleep better when you're relatively cool. It also prevents a spike in insulin, which is created by the pancreas to lower blood sugar. Insulin spikes counter the body's natural ability to produce growth hormone, which it normally makes most abundantly roughly an hour after falling asleep and in deep sleep stages. Additionally, high blood sugar early in sleep causes low blood sugar later in the night as the result of insulin release; our adrenal response and the break in our parasympathetic nervous system then rouses us from sleep.

- *Don't exercise late.* Don't exercise vigorously too close to bedtime; exercising earlier in the day, however, is great and can contribute to a good night's sleep.

- *Eliminate blue light.* While most light can affect one's ability to fall asleep by reducing the amount of melatonin (a sleep-inducing hormone) produced by the pineal gland, blue light (e.g., from screens such as TVs, laptops, phones, and tablets) has the strongest effect. So, eliminate "blue" light in your bedroom before you go to sleep. Interestingly, candlelight, especially certain scented candles, is fine and may actually promote sleep. Whether it is the light itself or the fact that it is coming from a stimulating TV show or irritating email, turning off the blue light can only contribute to sleep.

- *Reduce late-night caffeine.* Refrain from drinking caffeine and limit alcohol in the hours before bed. Everyone is different, and a glass of wine with dinner probably won't hurt your sleep, but having a few or more drinks may make you sleepy (and a lot of drinks may cause you to pass out in an alcoholic haze). They will play havoc with your sleeping system later in the night; you'll have similar insulin/blood sugar reactions to having food before bed, but worse.

- *Adhere to a regular sleeping/waking schedule.* Our bodies operate on what is called a circadian rhythm, which includes an established and regular sleep and wake time that, like your stomach preparing for its regular meal (mobilizing digestive juices and perhaps even growling), makes it easier on the body when adhered to. Not adhering to this regular schedule makes it harder to obtain the ideal amount and quality of sleep.

- *Incorporate meditation.* Try to shut down your thoughts—especially your worries—before bed. Meditation is good for this purpose, but simply clearing your mind is fine. Writing down the "worries" or chores before sleep frees the mind to let go of the never-ending loop in short-term memory that bugs us about an important matter. Also, avoid watching, reading, or discussing anything that upsets or angers you right before bed.

- *Control your environment.* Keep the bedroom cool, quiet, and dark. Studies show we can fall asleep faster and more deeply by moving from a relatively warmer environment to a cooler one. Too much light can reduce melatonin production and even initiate the process of daily awakening, and of course, noise—other than "white noises" that can be used to block the perception of other disruptive noises—can disrupt the quality and quantity of sleep.

- *Be cautious about sleeping pills.* Yes, they do make you sleepy, especially ones containing antihistamines, which most over-the-counter sleeping pills do. "Z" types (referred to as such because the generic names contain the letter "z") such as eszopiclone (Lunesta) and zolpidem (Ambien) are helpful for falling asleep, but these pills all have side effects and other drawbacks, and are not designed to help you stay asleep. While benzodiazepines like Valium, Klonopin, Ativan, and Xanax facilitate falling and staying asleep, this class of drug should only be taken on a one-time, "emergency" basis. Benzos act on similar GABA receptors in the brain as alcohol and progesterone, but it is believed these drugs also have their own receptors. They do relieve anxiety and may make it easier to sleep for a while, but they affect sleep architecture negatively, diminishing the quantity of sleep at each stage. Just as troubling, they are highly addictive. Unless you are among the roughly 15 percent of the population that can use benzodiazepines without serious side effects, don't use them regularly as a sleep aid. Benzodiazepines may soon be identified as the next silent scourge after opiate and opioid addiction, with much longer withdrawal periods and long-term side effects. They are certainly not a long-term solution to insomnia or useful for sleep apnea. And, while they may lead you to believe you slept better, their effect to relax the body invariably exacerbates obstructive sleep apnea.

NOT-SO-OBVIOUS SLEEP HELPERS

Beyond the basics, here are some additional suggestions that may facilitate a good night's rest:

- *Take a hot bath or shower.* Twenty minutes before bed, get into a hot bath, shower, or get into a home sauna. As mentioned, the move from hot to cold helps reduce body temperature and puts you into a sleep mode. You may also consider purchasing a bed-cooling system. Many types exist at various price points, but they all help create a cool environment that promotes sleep. Because I like to sleep in a cold room and my wife does not, I bought a cooling system that reduces the temperature only on my side of the bed.

- *Consider CBD.* While observing proper sleep hygiene is the best way to obtain a good night's rest, supplemental products may help. As most people know, cannabidiol is one of the active ingredients in cannabis (separate and distinct from THC, which is psychoactive) and is being used for a wide range of health purposes—some valid, some not. Some studies have suggested its ability to reduce anxiety can help people under excessive stress sleep better, though whether this ability is sustainable over the long term is an open question. The recommended dosages are between 25 and 175 mg before bedtime. Adding THC, the psychoactive component of cannabis, is initially not recommended in combination with CBD for sleep. THC tends to be "activating" rather than "sedating" for most people, although some studies and many anecdotal reports note that combining a smaller fraction of THC with CBD can treat insomnia more effectively.

- *Try progesterone.* Contrary to what you might think, this steroid hormone is present in both men and women; both sexes produce small amounts in their adrenal glands and gonads (testes in males and ovaries in females), though women produce much more in their ovaries. As we age, we produce less of this hormone. Progesterone has a soothing effect on our bodies, acting on our brain's GABA receptors as a calming neurotransmitter. It's been found to help us not only fall asleep, but stay asleep. You do need a prescription for progesterone. Progesterone taken orally is better than other delivery methods (transdermal, IV, nasal, subcutaneous) because orally it converts to dihydroprogesterone and 5-allopregnanolone more readily and both metabolites are more effective at agonizing (activating) GABA receptors. However, those individuals taking finasteride (brand names Propecia and Proscar) will not enjoy the same benefits because the enzyme blocked by finasteride is needed to convert progesterone to the aforementioned metabolites.

- *Experiment with naps.* In some cultures, naps or siestas are an accepted routine and they help people restart their day with renewed energy. The conventional wisdom is that short naps—fifteen to twenty minutes—won't do any harm and may re-energize us. While we still need more studies to determine the true efficacy of naps, be aware that sleep pressure builds throughout the day because of our circadian rhythms, and the result of all that pressure is that we're ready to sleep at our usual bedtime. If we interrupt that pressure with naps—especially overlong naps—then we may be decreasing this pressure and making it more difficult to fall asleep at night. Still, some people don't get enough sleep at night and it's possible that making up for that deficit during the day can help. Theoretically, the best length for this "makeup" nap is ninety minutes—the amount of time necessary to go through all the stages of sleep.

- *Prioritize sleep.* Recognize that if you're an athlete, getting adequate sleep is just as important as a good workout. Perhaps it's the workout warriors' sense of invulnerability that's the problem, but as I noted earlier, I see people in great shape who often don't get enough sleep. This is a *huge* mistake. During the day, we exercise hard and our sympathetic nerve system is operating, often using glycogen in our muscles for energy purposes. At night when we sleep, our parasympathetic nervous system takes over and embarks on the rest, repair, and replenishment of cells and tissue we've broken down. Without sufficient sleep, you're likely to overtrain and injure yourself while working out.

Why Exercise May Be the Single Most Important "Cheat"

AS WITH DIET and nutrition, no single exercise regimen fits everyone. For some people, brisk thirty-minute walks daily are sufficient. For others, two-a-day morning high-intensity interval training sessions followed by afternoon cardio workouts are appropriate. To find the right type of exercise, you need to figure out what your goals are.

- Do you just want to maintain a base level of physical fitness?
- Do you want to lose weight?
- Do you want to develop six-pack abs or be a bodybuilder?

Beyond goals, age is also a factor. Are you twenty-five or sixty-five? In addition, some people are attempting to recover from an injury or illness and need an exercise routine that fits their rehab requirements. Others are training for a particular event, such as a marathon, and they need to build their fitness levels.

Therefore, my exercise recommendations will vary with these and other factors. I will, however, make certain recommendations tied to healthspan, which can serve as foundational elements for whatever exercise program you choose. One certainty is that exercise is essential for healthspan. I call it: "the great equalizer."

THE AEROBIC VERSUS ANAEROBIC CALORIE EFFICIENCY ADVANTAGE

Most people are aware that exercise offers many benefits, including decreasing the risks of cardiovascular mortality, diabetes, certain types of cancer, osteoporosis, and mood disorders. From getting a better night's sleep to helping us live longer, the benefits are varied and significant. As mentioned, exercise can even be used to compensate for bad habits that include not getting enough sleep—at least where it involves the disruption to insulin sensitivity.

While many types of exercise can help you obtain at least some of these benefits, one specific approach is particularly valuable. To help you understand its value, let's examine the physiological differences between aerobic and anaerobic exercise. Aerobic exercise uses oxygen to produce energy in the cell, while anaerobic exercise produces energy without using oxygen.

CELLULAR RESPIRATION

CHEMICAL ENERGY O_2

GLYCOLYSIS
GLUCOSE → PYRUVIC ACID

KREBS CYCLE

ELECTRON (HYDROGEN) TRANSPORT SYSTEM

2 ATP

CO_2

36 ATP

H_2O

Aerobic Energy Production
1 kilocalorie yields 38 ATP (energy units usable by the body)

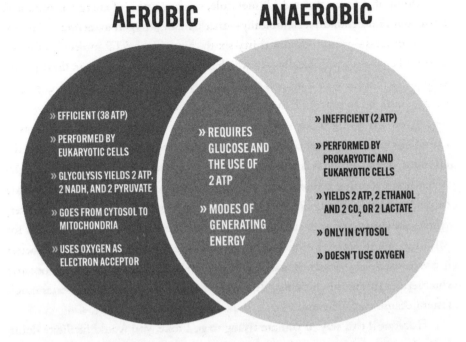

AEROBIC   ANAEROBIC

AEROBIC
» EFFICIENT (38 ATP)
» PERFORMED BY EUKARYOTIC CELLS
» GLYCOLYSIS YIELDS 2 ATP, 2 NADH, AND 2 PYRUVATE
» GOES FROM CYTOSOL TO MITOCHONDRIA
» USES OXYGEN AS ELECTRON ACCEPTOR

SHARED
» REQUIRES GLUCOSE AND THE USE OF 2 ATP
» MODES OF GENERATING ENERGY

ANAEROBIC
» INEFFICIENT (2 ATP)
» PERFORMED BY PROKARYOTIC AND EUKARYOTIC CELLS
» YIELDS 2 ATP, 2 ETHANOL AND 2 CO_2 OR 2 LACTATE
» ONLY IN CYTOSOL
» DOESN'T USE OXYGEN

	AEROBIC RESPIRATION	**ANAEROBIC RESPIRATION**
STAGES	GLYCOLYSIS LINK REACTION THE KREBS CYCLE OXIDATIVE PHOSPHORYLATION	GLYCOLYSIS FERMENTATION
OXIDATION OF GLUCOSE	COMPLETE	INCOMPLETE
TOTAL ATP PRODUCED	HIGH (~36)	LOW (2)
LOCATION	CYTOPLASM AND MITOCHONDRIA	CYTOPLASM
PRODUCTS	CO_2, H_2O	YEAST: CO_2, ETHANOL MAMMALS: LACTATE

Similarities and Differences in Aerobic versus Anaerobic Energy Production

Think of it this way: an ATP molecule, the basic unit of energy, is produced in the cell's mitochondria. Aerobically—that is, using oxygen to facilitate the conversion process—we can obtain thirty-six to thirty-eight ATP molecules for one calorie of energy. Anaerobically—in which the cell doesn't use oxygen for this conversion but instead uses a process called glycolysis (involving muscle glycogen)—we produce two to four ATP molecules for one calorie of energy.

If you are trying to lose fat, it may seem as if aerobics is a superior form of exercise since it creates much more ATP for every energy calorie. In fact, just the opposite is true. While it is true that we tend to use fat for energy more than glycogen when training aerobically (typically "Zone 2" or below—i.e., below lactate threshold, or below that point at which it starts getting difficult to talk while exercising), you would have to exercise for an inordinate amount of time each day for this to be your primary fat loss tool. If you're trying to lose weight, it's much better to use calories inefficiently. It takes a long time to burn calories aerobically because you are using them so efficiently. The anaerobic process gets rid of calories much faster because it's inefficient.

Think of it this way: if you are trying to go broke, you would facilitate doing so by paying more money for something than it is worth, say twice its price/value. In the case of anaerobic versus aerobic calorie expenditure, one is "paying" approximately ten to twenty times the price in calories using the anaerobic versus the aerobic system.

THE ANAEROBIC MUSCLE-BUILDING ADVANTAGE

Just as important, anaerobic exercise builds muscle, which provides our bodies with functional ability and a certain look. Building muscle also helps us maintain our metabolism, which means that we burn more calories, not just when we exercise but hours later. I bet you've never heard one of your buddies ribbing you with, "Hey pal, you really missed it. Last night, we went to the library and studied Einstein's general theory of relativity, and whew, we must have burned at least 2,000 calories!" No, that's in part, because the average human brain requires about 300 calories per day, and if you really increase your mental activity, you may burn an additional 20 calories per day.

The main reason we have to eat as much food as we do is to support our muscle mass; not just while actively using it, but maintaining it on our skeleton. So, adding muscle comes at an increased caloric cost, requiring and burning more calories. Anaerobic exercise has an "afterburn" effect that helps us burn calories long after we stop working out. Just keeping that muscle on our frame requires more calories to maintain, so that we are literally burning more calories asleep than we would without that muscle. Further, we burn more calories carrying that muscle doing just our everyday tasks than we would without it.

That said, cardiovascular fitness is also important. Studies show that a good VO_2 max level—a cardiopulmonary-fitness measure showing how well your body sends oxygen to muscles—has a positive effect on longevity. Therefore, incorporating the aerobic use of energy ("cardio") into an anaerobic exercise routine is a good idea.

THE HIGH-INTENSITY INTERVAL TRAINING ADVANTAGE

While there is an association between healthspan and VO_2 max, so, too, is there a connection between muscle mass, muscle strength, and longevity, with strength being more important than muscle mass. So, our exercise regimen should include ways to develop both the aerobic and anaerobic energy systems. Exercise training that involves high intensity—higher than "cardio" or aerobic exercise and involving the anaerobic energy system—is required to stimulate muscle mass and strength accretion. Some people do aerobic activities such as jogging or swimming on certain days and anaerobic workouts on others, or they do aerobic in the morning and anaerobic in the afternoon. That's fine, but the two can also be combined in high-intensity interval training (HIIT). If you're not familiar with this term, it describes workouts that alternate intense exercise with rests or "active recovery" like slow walking on a treadmill, not to be confused with an entire workout dedicated to active recovery. Many different types of HIIT routines exist: incorporating kettlebells, weights, sprinting, ropes, and exercise bikes. As the name implies, the key is the *amount* (high) of intensity with which you train.

HIIT requires much less time than traditional cardio-only exercise routines—as little as fifteen minutes. These routines also tend to exert less wear and tear on joints because of their relatively short duration, though they may be harder on joints than a run or a walk for that short period. Studies show HIIT practitioners burn calories for several hours after the workout is completed and, because HIIT has a positive impact on metabolism through increased muscle accretion, they even burn calories during sleep.

Some people worry that HIIT will cause them to become muscle bound, but in reality it's difficult to create the type of body that serious weightlifters possess. Unless you're doing extreme HIIT, doing a lot of weightlifting, getting adequate rest, and drinking protein shakes like they're water, you probably won't become bulky. Keeping muscles supple and long through use of stretching techniques certainly makes them more functional and less likely to feel binding.

HIIT is also beneficial if you want to lose fat while continuing your aerobic routines, what I refer to as long, slow distance (LSD) exercise. You'll end up burning more calories during your run or bike ride because you've added muscle through HIIT and therefore are burning calories less efficiently. The adage, "It's better to teach a man to fish so he can eat for the rest of his life than give him a fish to eat" is apt. Because you are promoting the accretion of muscle mass, HIIT essentially requires your body to burn more calories, whether you're exercising aerobically, walking to the store, or sleeping.

A simple example: You are trying to burn 500 calories a day exercising. You spend an hour each day training aerobically on the bicycle doing so. Then, you decide to burn 500 calories a day weight lifting at high intensity. Either way, you burn your daily goal of 500 calories. Eventually, with the weight lifting (along with proper rest and nutrition), you add 5 percent of your body weight in muscle mass. Then, just by being alive and doing nothing else but fogging a mirror, you are burning more calories to maintain that muscle mass. In addition, whenever you perform any exercise—the same hour of exercise biking or weight lifting—you are burning not just 500 calories as before, but maybe 700 calories, because you are now carrying around that extra muscle (read: extra caloric demand), having taught your body to fish rather than giving it a fish every day. In this example, which can be modified upward in terms of muscle and daily caloric output, conceivably you would have accumulated enough muscle that on your day off, you burn that same daily goal of 500 calories without even exercising!

Still, recognizing that some people refuse to give up their aerobic exercise routines, I recommend at least alternating aerobic and anaerobic days. This can be effective if you reach the *aerobic threshold*, the point where your body begins to switch from the aerobic system of burning calories to the anaerobic one. You reach that point when you're working out aerobically and your body can no longer produce energy using oxygen, therefore it must switch to the inefficient method of glycolysis. By the way, this is not a hard transition line but gradations of one system over the other.

The trick, though, is making sure you reach this threshold, which isn't always easy to do. As you become more fit (and more efficient with calories), your body uses oxygen better, and it takes longer to reach the threshold. It therefore becomes harder (less efficient) to lose fat, as your body is more efficient at using calories aerobically during exercise. Therefore, in trying to lose fat, if you decide to alternate aerobic and anaerobic exercise, improve your cardiovascular fitness—as measured in part by this energy efficiency—slowly. It's better to be efficient with your time and inefficient with the way you burn calories.

Think about the difference between sprinters and long-distance runners. The former have well-defined muscles because they're engaging in an HIIT activity, while long-distance runners are doing an aerobic activity. Though many long-distance runners look thin, they actually are often carrying a good deal of fat, since they're not stimulating muscle growth. In fact, when people are struggling to put on weight, I suggest they begin to do aerobic exercises because this will make them more efficient with their calories and eventually help them add mass more easily once they begin to incorporate HIIT.

THE FLEXIBILITY ADVANTAGE

One area often neglected in the exercise component of healthspan is flexibility. Maintenance of functional movement not only requires strength but flexibility, and both combine to permit free and effective movement. Studies show that as we lose this facility, our quality of life and longevity decline. The very definition of life itself includes "movement" and, without this ability, our health suffers demonstrably and quickly. So, an exercise routine that incorporates compound movements—those that use multiple muscles rather than one muscle in isolation, thereby better duplicating natural and functional movement—as well as stretching is ideal to maintain and improve healthspan.

While all this may seem overwhelming to many who have not concentrated on exercise during one's life, there is help available for getting started. Personal trainers are now available in almost every gym; yoga and Pilates instructors are also often found there, or in their own studios, to help initiate and further guide would-be exercisers.

A word of caution, however: as with any profession, there are good and bad practitioners. One must *always* perform sufficient due diligence in selecting a trainer/instructor. There are organizations that certify trainers such as the National Academy of Sports Medicine and the American College of Sports Medicine, which provide some assurance that an individual has received adequate basic instruction in the principles of exercise physiology and weight training. The same applies to Pilates (the Pilates Method Alliance and the National Pilates Certification Program) as well as yoga (the Yoga Alliance and their Registered Yoga Teachers) organizations that certify their instructors with basic knowledge of their craft. Beyond certifications, it is wise to interview an individual as one would for any job hire to inquire about their training philosophy, gauge their demeanor, evaluate their listening skills, and assess whether they appear to practice what they preach.

Whatever your preference is—to lose fat, gain muscle, improve VO_2 max, or functional threshold power (on a bicycle)—exercise is probably the most important and powerful aspect of anyone's ambition to improve healthspan, especially since you have the most control over doing it daily. In addition to the areas of health mentioned above, one's functional abilities to move, to sit, to carry, to bend over, and to rise from the floor all affect one's healthspan. The adage "use or lose it" should not only be remembered but also proactively applied in determining one's exercise routine.

THE SEXY ADVANTAGE

The good news is, we now have an increased understanding of the critical impact that nutrition and exercise have on mitochondrial function. For example, we know that regular exercise is crucial for mitochondrial health. An overabundant intake of high-calorie, high-glycemic-load (carbohydrate) foods can injure mitochondrial performance, expressed by such disease pathologies as metabolic syndrome and diabetes, which are known detractors from sexual health, particularly erectile dysfunction and neurological function.

Therefore, a focus on exercise and nutrition helps us address sexual health challenges in a fresh and effective manner. Additionally, measuring endocrine (hormone) levels puts us in a position to learn if there are any acute deficiencies or over-expressions that may hurt sexual health. Optimizing what we eat and how we exercise, along with hormone replacement, can have a very beneficial effect on not just how we feel, but how we perform sexually. For example, blood tests that measure testosterone, estradiol (an estrogen), dihydrotestosterone, prolactin, luteinizing hormone, and follicle-stimulating hormone can offer tremendous insight as to whether hormone replacement is the correct intervention for improving both sexual and metabolic health.

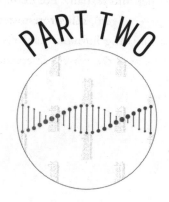

PART TWO

Aging with the Regenerative Advantage

Turning Back Time with Stem and Muse Cells

AS AN ATHLETE who has endured many injuries and has had to recover from more than twenty (closer to thirty) surgeries, I relish how stem and Muse cells rejuvenate the body. As a physician, I am gratified to use stem cell therapies on behalf of my patients to treat acute trauma or as preventive. Stem and Muse cells represent what regenerative medicine is all about—restoring the body from its roots or reversing the degeneration that occurs with the process of life and aging.

Before I delve deep into the science of stem and Muse cells—and I mean deep enough for my fellow nerds—let me highlight what is genuinely possible from a regenerative perspective with this longevity tool. I have treated and observed many patients who have benefited greatly from stem cell infusions. One of the first was a thirty-six-year-old athlete whom our clinic treated with stem cells (when it was legal, prior to the FDA white paper). He had extensively damaged his shoulders because of his athletic activities and, as a result, both shoulders had enormous amounts of inflammation, producing so much fluid that it was migrating into his neck. After draining his shoulders and extracting mesenchymal stem cells from his body fat, we injected seventy to eighty million stem cells to begin repairing the extensive damage. Ten days later, his condition improved so much that he was back to doing ten to twelve repetitions of 275-pound military presses (lifting weight overhead). The change was fast, dramatic, and provided early evidence that stem cells are highly effective against inflammation.

Another patient of mine is a middle-aged, self-made, very financially successful man who also always maintained his physical health until a doctor's prescribing error led to congestive heart failure with an ejection fraction of 12 percent. (Typically, a healthy heart ejects between 55 to 65 percent of the blood in the left ventricle out to the body at each beat; an ejection fraction of 12 percent is close to being incompatible with life.) He had the "world as his oyster" in almost every way except for his health; he was unable to play with his kids, maintain a sexually active marriage, exercise as he always had at the gym, or climb stairs without getting severely winded. After one intravenous infusion of approximately 150 million allogeneic (i.e., umbilical cord tissue–derived) stem cells, the patient recovered his heart function so that he could resume all the prior activities he had enjoyed in life prior to his heart injury, and his ejection fraction returned to 55 percent.

I recovered in similarly dramatic fashion after I had a nine-hour, eight-level (referring to the number of spinal vertebral discs) spine surgery that left me shuffling around like an infirm, elderly person. Acquaintances later told me that I appeared so hobbled and miserable that they were afraid to approach me. A stranger actually stopped me as I was shuffling down the street and asked if he should call an ambulance for me. I treated myself by injecting around 120 million mesenchymal stem cells (once stem cells are injected, they replicate, so the actual number doing the repair work is actually many more than the number injected). In less than a week, I was standing up straight, walking normally, and running on a treadmill.

These are just three of the many cases I can cite when it comes to stem cells and their role in helping to extend mobility and vitality during our race against aging. However, what is particularly interesting is what happened to those 120 million cells before they were intravenously infused. Let me provide you with the science that made these results, and makes many more, possible.

WHAT ARE STEM CELLS AND HOW DO THEY WORK TO RESTORE THE BODY?

From the Latin *regenerativus*, the idea of restoring the body is part of every major cultural and religious myth throughout recorded history. Nature, too, provides us with inspiration; think about a salamander who can regenerate a lost tail in a week's time. However, it wasn't until 1938 that scientists became adept at culturing cells, making it possible to replace organs and tissues. The first successful long-term kidney transplant in 1954 and the first heart transplant in 1967 represent regenerative medicine's pioneering efforts even though the term would not come into use until the late 1990s.

Today, stem and Muse cells are regenerative medicine's modern manifestations. Stem cells are not just being used for repairing joints, muscle, tendons, and ligaments, but also to restore metabolic health, cognitive well-being, and enhancing immune function. As the uses of stem cells continue to expand and safety and efficacy are better understood, underlying services such as long-term storage and banking of cells are beginning to become more available. Storage and banking services expand the opportunities to lock in your cells' biological age and eliminate the waiting time before treatment with your own cells when you need it.

Let's begin by defining what these cells are.

THE FIVE MAJOR CLASSES OF STEM CELLS

Cells are the basic building blocks of the body, but we possess a range of cell types with different purposes and abilities. Unlike other cells, stem cells can multiply like proverbial rabbits, thereby providing a great reservoir of new cells for our body as we grow while replacing ones that are damaged. Even better, some stem cells possess the ability to take the form of any specific cell as they divide. Thus, *stem cell* is an umbrella term, actually referring to five major classes of cells:

- *Unipotent*: one homogeneous type of stem cell
- *Oligopotent*: can differentiate (change) into a few different types of cells
- *Multipotent*: can differentiate into a closely related family of cells
- *Pluripotent*: can differentiate into almost any type of cell; embryonic cells are in this class
- *Totipotent*: can differentiate into any and all cell types and are the initial cells that form an embryo and give rise to pluripotent cells of the embryo

Stem cells are derived from our own tissues (autologous) or from a donated source (allogeneic). Donated embryonic or fetal cells have been the subject of considerable regulatory and ethical controversy, making them difficult to obtain unless you're enrolled in a study or receiving them as part of an Investigational New Drug program like those currently underway through American CryoStem and some other companies determined to get FDA approval for their use in the US.

One of the more practically effective forms of multipotent stem cells are called mesenchymal stem cells. They come from bone and fat in adults or from donated umbilical cord blood and can be used to address cardiac disease, joint injuries, and autoimmune disorders. Crucially, they can differentiate into bone, cartilage, and muscle cells and are often injected locally to address acute injury, such as a ligament sprain, using ultrasound-guided injection.

Last, there are Muse (multilineage differentiating stress-enduring) cells. Discovered in Japan in 2010, these pluripotent cells are even safer, insofar that they cannot be transformed into cancerous cells, which is a very small risk associated with certain stem cell therapies; they can cross the blood–brain barrier, making them an appropriate therapy for cognitive disorders and brain injuries. Additionally, donated Muse cells can be replicated much more quickly than other types, offering an expedited healing effect given that many more of these stem cells can be introduced at each therapy session. Conveniently obtained from fat cells, they are also cheaper to create in the laboratory—$1,000 per 300 million cells—than conventional stem cell therapies, which fall in the $5,000 to $20,000 range. Note that this does not include the cost of extraction via liposuction—$1,000 for a simple extraction to over $50,000 for a high-definition cosmetic liposuction—or the expense of cell infusion and/or injection, which can range from $200 to over $8,000 depending upon the physician's fee schedule. The higher-priced procedures tend to include more tangential considerations that are not necessary and do not affect the outcome, so I recommend shopping around. While Muse cells are a relatively new discovery, their benefits and safety make them the likely stem cell of choice in the future.

The rest of the chapter will explain these various types of stem cells in more detail and how they can be used to treat specific disorders and diseases.

HOW STEM CELLS WORK TO RESTORE THE BODY

Stem cells are relatively easy to harvest, often from the patient's own body, and are often less expensive than traditional treatments such as joint replacements and chronic "conservative" management including physical therapy, cortisone or hyaluronic acid–derivative injections, and pharmacological treatments (e.g., NSAIDs and painkillers). They also made headlines during the coronavirus pandemic because studies have found them to be effective in treating COVID-19, something I'll discuss further later in this chapter.

The good news is: we're just beginning to understand all the potential uses of these cells including their positive impact on longevity.

The bad news is: if you ask your doctor for stem cell treatment, he may look at you in bewilderment. The FDA has erected significant barriers (some for good reason) between you and your ability to access cellular treatments. Fortunately, options exist that allow you to access stem cell treatment despite these difficulties, options that can make a huge difference in your healthspan, including high-quality foreign clinics and expanded US FDA programs such as compassionate care and right to try.

Earlier, I described five classes of stem cells. Let's dig a bit deeper into what each of these cells are and how they heal.

TOTIPOTENT & PLURIPOTENT

Embryonic.

As the name implies, these cells help embryos grow and develop into babies. Totipotent cells can morph into any one of more than two hundred types of cells in the human body and give rise to pluripotent cells. Pluripotent cells can develop further along three different lines—endoderm, mesoderm, and ectoderm—to become multipotent stem cells. Embryonic stem cells have been the object of controversy, since some people raised objections to the use of these cells for medical treatment on ethical grounds. As a result, many doctors and researchers in the US and elsewhere have been reluctant to harvest these cells for medical use. In addition, many doctors reject the use of all "stem cells" outright in the ignorant belief that they are all obtained from embryos.

Induced pluripotent stem cells (iPS).

These are pluripotent stem cells created in the laboratory via the introduction of embryonic genes usually carried by viruses into somatic cells (tissue-specific cells, such as a skin cell) that are removed from a human subject. They act closely enough to embryonic stem cells to be called pluripotent and they can be used therapeutically as well as in the laboratory to create models for treating various diseases. For example: in one laboratory model, we can use these induced cells to create lung tissue and introduce a pneumonia-causing bacteria, following up with a novel antibiotic tested for efficacy.

MULTIPOTENT

Adult stem cells.

Also called *somatic* (or tissue-specific) stem cells, these cells replace or repair damaged cells of particular types. For instance, hematopoietic or blood stem cells can only fix blood cells. *Multipotent* means that they are limited in their capacity to take different forms; they can only assume the form of a small family of cells within a given type. Historically, one of the most common medical uses of stem cells is to treat leukemia, a cancer in which these hematopoietic cells, which originate in the bone marrow, are abnormal. Hematopoietic stem cells are taken from a donor and given to the patient in a process known as allogeneic stem cell transplant to help restore bone marrow harmed by chemotherapy.

Many types of adult stem cells exist, typically classified by their derivative source. It was previously thought that their respective functions were also strictly limited by their source, but recent studies show this not to be the case—some neural stem cells can differentiate into immune system cells. In addition, mesenchymal stem cells are those found in the stroma (connective tissue) surrounding various organs and tissues and, depending upon the origin, appear to have various capacities for differentiation and function. In short, it appears that even some of the stem cells we thought were less potent, and therefore restricted in their potential to repair, are able to change into a multitude of beneficial cells.

Certain types of stem cells can be found in specific areas of the body and not in others; the same type of stem cell can function in different ways depending on where in the body they're located. Bone marrow contains three types of stem cells: hematopoietic, endothelial, and mesenchymal. Mesenchymal stem cells found in fat's perivasculature (the blood vessels in and around it) behave differently than the mesenchymal stem cells harvested from bone marrow. As we'll see, certain types of stem cells from particular parts of the body are more effective for specific conditions.

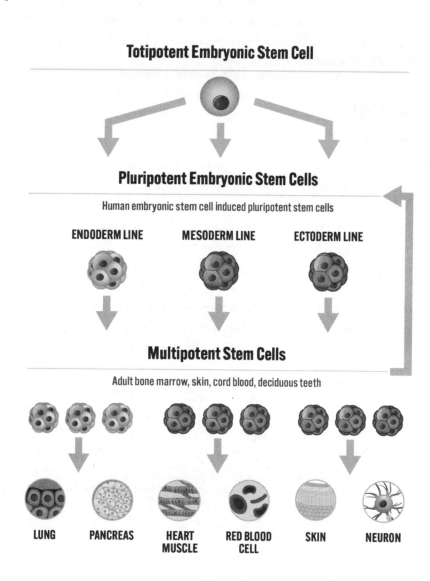

KNOWING THE DIFFERENCE BETWEEN
ALLOGENEIC AND AUTOLOGOUS CELLS

You'll recall that I defined the terms *allogeneic* (from donors) and *autologous* (from your own body) stem cells earlier. Now, let's examine the positives and negatives depending on the source of the cells.

When using allogeneic cells, you don't have to endure harvesting stem cells from your own tissues, since they come from donors. Until recently, these cells have been obtained from blood or bone marrow of qualified and screened donors. More recently, mesenchymal stem cells harvested from donated umbilical cord tissue are being used for allogeneic stem cell treatments. This is an advantage for those that do not have time to go through the harvesting process or cannot because of injury or for other reasons. For instance, if you've had a brain injury, you will need treatment within seventy-two hours, but stem cells usually require at least three to four weeks to harvest, process, and "expand" (the term used for replicating the number of stem cells in the lab). This makes a case for harvesting one's own cells proactively in order to have them "banked" in case of need in the future. American CryoStem has presented to the NFL the science of and ability to treat concussions immediately using players' harvested stem cells, preventing any long-term damage.

You may also prefer allogeneic cells because you're thin and you lack sufficient fat from which stem cells are drawn. You may not want or be able to undergo a bone marrow "tap" (aspiration, meaning drawing through a needle into a syringe); the hip is used to access the bone marrow and collect stem cells. Bone marrow aspirations can make you feel like you fell off your bike and landed on your hip, but the real problem is that the number of cells that can be harvested can vary and is limited in both quantity and types. With bone marrow aspirations, the mix of three stem cells types (endothelial, mesenchymal, and hematopoietic) may serve better than just mesenchymal, but these aspirated stem cells cannot be expanded in the lab to produce even more, which may be useful, if not necessary. Further, you may be physically unable to tolerate the procedure.

In these cases, having autologous stem cells stored, or donated allogeneic stem cells can be a game changer.

An allogeneic procedure may also be necessary because the use of umbilical cord *tissue-derived* mesenchymal stem cells is not yet FDA approved. Umbilical cord, *blood-derived* stem cells are FDA approved, but with significant limitations that restrict its use to "allogeneic hematopoietic cell transplantations appropriate for patients suffering from a blood or immune cell disorder."[11] One downside to this allogeneic model is if you require additional treatment(s) over time, there is no assurance that you can receive cells from the same donor or manufacturing batch, and the matched cells from the first treatment may not be available for future treatments. This increases the risks of rejection or the complications in finding an appropriately matched donor sample.

Stem cells harvested via the autologous method have the advantage of being from your own body rather than from other people, where the (very rare) risk of rejection or disease exists despite extensive screening. Doctors harvest cells from the patient, process and expand them, then return them in curative forms to the patient. Certain cell sources such as adipose tissue can be collected, processed, expanded, and banked for future use.

The process begins with the removal of approximately 2 to 4 ounces (25 to 50 mL) of tissue from which billions of your own genetically matched cells can be created and stored for future "on demand" access. This would specifically appeal to patients with chronic conditions and diseases such as arthritis or multiple sclerosis, where ongoing cell therapies (one or two per year) are the optimal treatment. Using a banking strategy is important for reducing secondary health risks and additional costs associated with cell harvesting for each treatment when developing a long-term cellular therapy plan for disease mitigation, regenerative therapy, and wellness treatments. The ability to have banked samples of your own cells readily available will reduce the average cost of each treatment and eliminate the opportunities for cell rejection or graft versus host disease, the most serious potential side effects that can result from using donor cells.

In addition, it appears that one's own stem cells will actually engraft, meaning they will target somatic cells in need of repair and differentiate themselves to become the needed somatic cell. This isn't always the case with the allogeneic method, which employs a different technique to achieve a similar result. In the case of an allogeneic stem cell, it appears that it acts as a "placeholder" for a patient's own cell that is made in the bone marrow after receiving a signal (RNA) from the accompanying cells harvested from allogeneic sources. Along with stem cells, other biologically active components are harvested and are an integral part of the regenerative process.

THE HISTORY AND FUTURE OF MUSE CELLS

To be thorough in the explanation of stem cells and their benefit, I must also include a discussion around Muse cells. Muse cells were discovered accidentally by Dr. Mari Dezawa, who has been credited with the discovery at Japan's Tohoku University. According to Dr. Dezawa, she was working in her lab on a hot summer afternoon when she received an invitation to a wine party that evening. In her haste to finish her work so she could attend the party, she made a mistake. As a result of adding a trypsin solution instead of a culture medium to the culture dish, she created a harsh, nutrient-devoid environment that severely stressed the cells in the culture. Examining the results of her failed experiment, she discovered "stress-enduring" pluripotent cells.

A doctor with whom I work, UCLA's Dr. Gregorio Chazenbalk, was also part of this discovery process. He was doing an after-hours experiment with cells at a UCLA lab and the centrifuge he was using failed mid-experiment conduction. So, without cleaning up, he broke for dinner. When he returned the next morning, he found that Muse cells had grown in his absence. By ignoring them and, more specifically, by making their environment more hostile, he had put the cells under extreme stress, which served as a catalyst for their formation. As stress-enduring cells, they appear to reside in stroma surrounding various tissues and organs and emerge as a final line of defense in keeping people alive. Dr. Chazenbalk created a procedure that placed a huge strain on mesenchymal cells culled from fat which has been highly effective in producing Muse cells.

Muse cells are the superstars of the cell universe. They are pluripotent, a quality that makes them versatile; they morph into whatever type of cells patients require, but they also possess advantages that stem cells lack.

First, they don't produce teratomas (cancerous cells). One of the fears people have about stem cells is that they can cause cancer. In reality, the likelihood of this happening is low for most types of stem cell treatments, except for nerve cells. We've found that when stem cells—not Muse cells—are injected into the spinal canal (e.g., to treat spinal cord injuries), they produce cancer cells about 25 percent of the time. Theoretically, this is because nerve cells are so complex and differentiated that more things can go wrong with them as opposed, for instance, to the simpler cells of the heart muscle. It is believed that this risk will drop or disappear as our technique for administering them is refined. The good news about Muse cells is that they don't have this issue.

Second, Muse cells can cross the blood–brain barrier. As I noted earlier, this is a major advantage when it comes to treating brain injuries, since they're the only type of stem cell capable of crossing this boundary, and thus can be administered intravenously rather than being injected directly into the brain. As a result, it's the right stem cell treatment option for diseases like Parkinson's, because it helps regenerate the brain cells that create dopamine, a key neurotransmitter essential for managing this disease.

Third, Muse cells are hardy, which means they replicate better, providing a greater quantity of cells and thus accelerating the healing process.

Fourth, they lack a "fingerprint," meaning that they can be taken from a donor and infused in a recipient without fear of rejection. With most other donated (allogeneic) stem cells, we screen people to confirm that donated cells are a close enough match for the recipient to accept, but this is an imperfect science and it can be difficult to assess a match.

Fifth, they're easily obtained from fat cells, though they're found all over the body.

Sixth, the cost of Muse cell treatment is less than stem cells, at least for now. At the research/academic level, it costs approximately $1,000 to obtain 300 million Muse cells. Of course, that may change over time as insurance companies get involved, but at the moment these superstar cells are available at a relative bargain rate.

A seventh benefit may concern longevity. My friend Bob Harding is a brilliant engineer who has been interested in "anti-aging" since the days of the field's pioneering Durk Pearson and Sandy Shaw; he's been "rolling his own" treatments for aging ever since, based upon his extensive culling of the existing research. He has coined a term for using Muse cells to increase healthspan: being able to *youthanize* our bodies. Given the negative connotations of the pre-existing term *euthanize*, I have my doubts about *youthanize*'s probability of catching on. However, it does describe what Muse cells may be able to accomplish.

Though it's going to require more research, the theory is that if we proactively infuse our bodies with Muse cells, they will be stored in the body until we need them. Then, if we're injured in some way, they will activate and repair damaged cells. Along with serving as a preventive bulwark for various diseases and disorders, Muse cells also may extend our youthful appearance and healing properties enabling us to look, feel, and function better. What is frustrating is that much of the research is documented in Japanese, and despite the treatments' proven efficacy and immense potential, very little work is being done to universally advance use of Muse cells. Certain countries that promote medical tourism, such as Costa Rica and Grand Cayman, provide these treatments as they do stem cell treatments. Currently, Dr. Chazenbalk is treating patients in Peru.

HOW STEM CELLS ARE BEING USED WORLDWIDE

Unfortunately, in the United States, stem and Muse cell treatments either are still viewed as "experimental" or invite skepticism, at least from some medical professionals. I've even had patients tell me their doctors are dismissive of stem cell procedures or are completely ignorant about how effectively they work. While there is good reason to be cautious—stem and Muse cell treatments are still in their relative infancy—there is also good reason to study them further and test therapeutic approaches. Both patients and many of us in the medical community have been frustrated by the FDA's cautious approach. The FDA issued an influential white paper on stem cells that effectively made it illegal for doctors to treat patients with stem cells, which is why—unless you are receiving stem cells for one of the few approved uses, like a bone marrow transplant—you have to participate in a trial, study, or go to another country to take advantage of this treatment.

OFF-LABEL STEM USE WITH PRP

Platelet-rich plasma (PRP) derived from one's own blood can be used to restore tissue sensitivity to both men and women. When combined with stem cells, this can have powerfully restorative effects on anatomical function. PRP was originally performed on men in an effort to restore erectile function and girth; an injection of PRP into the cavernosum of the penis—often with a dermal filler such as Juvederm injected into the crown of the penis—was invented and dubbed the Casanova Procedure by Dr. Roger Murray. When injected into the vagina and sometimes in and around the clitoris, the procedure is called the Cleopatra Procedure (a.k.a. the "O Shot").

The FDA's attitude is due partly to the actions of a small number of companies that have sought to take financial advantage of patients and offer stem cell "cures" that range from flawed to fraudulent. Many doctors and companies running stem cell programs, however, are scrupulously honest and diligent about ensuring they provide high-quality, effective treatments.

The total number of available studies has increased in the past decade as cell therapy manufacturers have responded to the FDA's requirement for clinical studies to determine safety, efficacy, dosage (number of cells in a single treatment), and frequency. Many of the most difficult diseases to treat such as multiple sclerosis, brain injuries or other neurologic conditions, osteoarthritis, muscular dystrophy, and other degenerative conditions will require multiple treatments over time and/or booster treatments across a patient's lifetime. Accessing available FDA studies can be very challenging, often requires travel to the treatment sites, and requires follow-up analysis and testing that can span months to years. These studies can also be used for FDA-approved alternative routes to treatment during a phase I safety study or following the completion of the safety study. These two main alternatives to actually participating in a study are compassionate use and right to try, both part of the FDA expanded-access programs. These opportunities warrant investigation by informed and interested patients seeking cellular therapies in the US for conditions currently under clinical study. Information can be found at clinicaltrials.gov for ongoing and new clinical studies that may be accessed through these expanded-use programs.

Clinicians in Germany, Japan, Taiwan, and other countries have used intravenous infusion of stem cells to repair damaged heart tissue as well as to treat arthritis, cancer, infertility, diabetes, and stroke (when there's damage to brain tissue). In the US, many doctors have focused on using stem cells to treat joint and musculoskeletal injuries. Because of legal restrictions and safety concerns, we have not capitalized on stem cell treatments as widely as other countries have. While it's obviously important to avoid harming patients, it's just as important to make effective treatments available to them. Also, the US religious right has discouraged the use of embryonic stem cells on the basis of faith-influenced ethical rhetoric, preventing greater access to these highly effective pluripotent cells for healing purposes.

Since the coronavirus pandemic, we've seen various hospitals and researchers testing the effectiveness of stem cells to treat COVID-19. A hospital in New York City experimented with giving mesenchymal stem cells to twelve infected patients on ventilators and, shortly after receiving the stem cell treatment, ten of them were able to be removed from breathing assistance. Regenerative medicine company

Mesoblast is conducting a three hundred-person trial to determine if stem cells can help COVID patients with lung inflammation.

There isn't enough space here to list all the conditions for which stem cells have been used successfully or all the different trials for treatments of other disorders and diseases. But, to give you a sense of the range of uses, let me spotlight a few significant areas:

- *Stroke.* The theory here is that, after a stroke, stem cells can replace damaged or destroyed cells and thereby restore impaired functions. A Stanford University study[12] documented how an infusion of stem cells helped restore speech and mobility for a young woman who required a wheelchair and couldn't talk after surviving a debilitating stroke. Muse cells may have particular relevance here because they, unlike other stem cells, are capable of crossing the blood–brain barrier.

- *Type 1 diabetes and other autoimmune diseases.* With these diseases, the body's immune system goes haywire and attacks healthy cells. Stem cells may be capable of repairing damaged cells and even resetting the immune system so it returns to normal and doesn't continue attacking the body's own cells. Several hospitals in the US currently offer autologous bone marrow cellular therapies for resetting the immune system following high-dose radiation and chemotherapy treatments in cancer patients.

- *Spinal cord issues.* In the past, people with severed or severely damaged spinal cords had little hope of regaining much function because destroyed nerves can't be repaired. Stem cells, however, may be able to replace these nerve cells and help restore leg and arm function.[13] A caveat: treatment must begin very soon after the injury occurs or motor function becomes much more difficult to restore. Much work still needs to be done in this area, but stem cells offer real promise as the basis of future treatments.

HARVESTING STEM CELLS FOR RESTORATIVE CARE

The many stem and Muse cell studies and trials currently underway, if successful, will increase pressure on regulatory and legislative bodies to make stem cell treatments more widely available and on insurance companies to cover most of the cost.

I should also emphasize that stem cell harvesting and treatment techniques are evolving; new methods may soon be developed that will supplant the ones discussed here. For now, though, common techniques for harvesting include aspiration—the previously described bone marrow "tapping." Another technique, apheresis, is a process by which catheterization and a centrifuge are used to extract the stem cells from blood. While not as painful as a bone marrow aspiration, the procedure is time consuming (usually four to six hours) and involves sitting with catheters in each arm while a machine draws blood from one arm, separates the white blood cells (those containing the stem cells) using a centrifuge, and then replaces the remainder via the opposite arm. An additional time burden is that, unlike aspiration, apheresis patients require injections of a granulocyte-macrophage colony-stimulating factor (GM-CSF), a drug that ramps up the body's production of stem cells, that must be performed daily for three to five days prior to apheresis in order to mobilize stem cells from the bone marrow into the blood for harvesting.

Yet another approach that currently has much broader applications and appeal in the stem cell community involves extracting mesenchymal stem cells from body fat through liposuction. As you'll recall, mesenchymal stem cells are multipotent, which is to say, limited in their capacity to differentiate into certain types of cells. But to scientists' surprise, recent research shows that the cells appear more flexibly mutable than previously thought. These cells don't have to come from a donor, but can be obtained autologously, ensuring that the cells will most likely engraft and greatly reducing the chance that they might be rejected or carry disease. Mesenchymal stem cells obtained from one's own fat provide a means to harvest and expand far more stem cells in the lab than other techniques and, along with allogeneic umbilical-derived mesenchymal cells, appear to be the most efficient and useful of all stem cells. Adding the opportunity to bank fat-derived stem cells for future use further supports their efficiency and usefulness for cellular therapies requiring multiple treatments over time or for wellness applications as we age.

STEM CELL SUCCESS STORIES

I started this chapter sharing a few success stories using stem cells from my own clinic. Now I'll share success stories from around the world.[14]

In China, a twenty-six-year-old man was diagnosed with type 1 diabetes. He was treated with amniotic membrane–derived stem cells from his infant son and, three months after treatment, he was no longer insulin dependent. For the next thirty-six months, his blood glucose levels were under control.[15]

Sara Hughes was a twenty-two-year-old woman who had been battling systemic juvenile idiopathic arthritis, an autoimmune disease, all her life. Despite many different types of treatments, she wasn't getting better. Then she discovered Dr. Stanley Jones, who ran a company in Mexico that provided stem cell treatments. Because of FDA regulations, she had to travel to Mexico to receive treatment. Shortly after, she began to recover from her disease in dramatic ways. Sara was able to eat food, rather than be fed through a tube. The hives and infections caused by the disease vanished. She also was able to stop the chemotherapy treatments and maintenance drugs that had been essential for keeping her disease from spiraling out of control.[16]

At the ThriveMD medical clinic in Denver, Colorado, a forty-six-year-old man received stem cells to treat both a back problem and a torn Achilles tendon. The clinic reported[17] that the patient was seeking to avoid spinal fusion surgery and heal his tendon. After having tried physical therapy, massage, and acupuncture and not obtaining significant improvement in his conditions, he underwent a stem cell procedure at ThriveMD. One month after treatment, the patient reported less pain as well as a greater ability to exercise. After one year, he was pain free and ran a marathon without his back or Achilles bothering him.

Twenty-one-year-old Kris Boesen was involved in a car accident that left him with a broken neck, initially completely paralyzed and on a ventilator to breathe. Eventually, he gained the ability to move his left arm up and down only, albeit with a clenched fist, yet he still had no use of his legs. After an injection of only ten million stem cells directly into his spinal cord, he now can lift weights, sign his name, operate his motorized wheelchair, and feed himself.[18] Part of the success with Kris derives from relatively early treatment and his age. We have animal studies showing that brain lesions caused by trauma can be 100 percent reversed and cured if stem cell treatment is given within seventy-two hours of initial injury. Why are more people like Kris not being treated in the hope and expectation that they could enjoy partial or complete resolution of damage caused by spinal cord injuries? Finding and getting permission for these treatments in the United States is still exceptionally hard because of the FDA's regulatory constraints.

HOW TO EXPLORE AND EXERCISE YOUR STEM/MUSE CELL OPTIONS

If you're like most people, you're excited about the possibilities of stem cell treatment, but the FDA has only approved it for a few conditions. As a result, you must scramble a bit to gain access. While a number of grassroots clinics have sprung up to provide this treatment, it's difficult to ascertain the quality of their cells, the effectiveness of their methods, or the safety of their methodologies. It is unwise to shop at the Stem Cells "R" Us store around the corner.

As noted earlier, your options boil down to the numerous stem cell trials being conducted in the US or the equally numerous clinics in other countries. To get started exploring these options, you can ask your doctor if they know of a trial in your area or a reputable clinic in another country. However, the odds are that your doctor will know less about this than you do after reading this book.

Here are the steps to follow in order to find the treatment that is right for you:

First, take advantage of websites that provide an overview of trials and clinics throughout the world. One of the best sites is run by the International Society for Stem Cell Research.[19] This site provides links to a wide range of other sites that may help you find what you're looking for in your area or in other countries. It also is filled with information about stem cells and conditions that experts deem treatable by this method. The University of California at San Francisco[20] and the Mayo Clinic[21] also have sites that provide information about stem cell trials.

Second, endeavor to match the particular type of stem cell treatment with your specific condition. Not only are there different types of stem cells; there are also different subtypes and ways of delivering the stem cells. If you have leukemia, for instance, you want the "standard" treatment—all three stem cell types collected via bone marrow aspiration or apheresis. But let's say you have worn knee cartilage or a partially torn meniscus; in this instance, autologous or allogeneic mesenchymal stem cells are preferable because they're more efficient and economical than the stem cells used in bone marrow transplants. Sometimes, the match also depends on feasibility. If you're thin with little body fat, it may be difficult if not impossible to extract stem cells from fat. Similarly, it may be necessary to obtain cells from a donor rather than from oneself, since the latter may increase the odds of a condition (such as cancer) returning.

Third, determine what you're willing and able to pay. Insurance won't cover anything except stem cells obtained through bone marrow transplants. The costs can run from free (certain trials) to quite expensive. Different methods have different costs, ranging from as "little" as $3,000 per treatment to approximately $20,000 (and more, given specific treatment types and patient needs) for a liposuction, stem cell harvesting, processing, and expansion to obtain one's first 150 million autologous adipose-derived mesenchymal stem cells. In many cases, liposuction is the most cost-effective option for obtaining autologous mesenchymal stem cells, which can be multiplied in the lab readily, offering more bang for the buck.

Fourth, assess geographically where your treatment is available. If you have multiple sclerosis, the effective treatment is with infused adipose-autologous mesenchymal stem cells, but this isn't available in the US. As mentioned earlier, one of my patients with MS found a terrific source for this treatment in the Cayman Islands, and immediately after receiving two infusions, he recovered significant vision and muscular coordination. Dr. Neil Riordan, who runs the Stem Cell Institute in Panama, has an excellent reputation, and his institute was one of the pioneers in stem cell treatments. Of course, in considering the place to go, cost is a factor.

Fifth, educate yourself about whether a given clinic/treatment has been the subject of lawsuits, controversy, or other negative publicity. The saying "A few bad apples spoil the whole barrel" applies. I have observed some stem cell purveyors exaggerating claims, taking shortcuts with their techniques, and engaging in other practices that are ethically dubious. Any hot healthcare field attracts some sketchy people. An educated consumer is the best defense against these individuals. Look for clinics run by people with strong science/medical credentials. Ask your doctor or other person with deep medical knowledge about the validity of their methods and stem cell extraction and infusion approaches. Beware of any clinic that is selling stem cells like late-night TV pitchmen hawking slicers-and-dicers: "50 PERCENT OFF 100 MILLION STEM CELLS FOR ONE WEEK ONLY! PLUS A FREE TOASTER!"

Sixth, track emerging treatment developments. Stem cells represent a rapidly evolving field, not just scientifically but from a regulatory perspective. Invariably, new and more effective treatments will emerge for a wide range of conditions, and just as invariably, stem cells will gain greater acceptance in different sectors of society. As I mentioned, I'm associated with a company called American CryoStem, and it is currently talking with representatives at Walter Reed Hospital and the National Institutes of Health about conducting government-funded stem cell studies. But this is only one of countless studies that are being undertaken, and by regularly checking sites such as the International Society for Stem Cell Research (www.isscr.org), or www.clinicaltrials.gov, you can keep abreast of developments and better determine which ones might be relevant to your particular condition.

Once these studies are approved and funded, doctors like me will recruit appropriate patients and administer stem cell treatments, conclude studies, and publish results. Well-funded, high-profile studies of successful therapies will spread the word and help stem cells gain acceptance.

THE CASE FOR BANKING YOUR STEM CELLS NOW

As promising as stem cell treatments are, they are not a panacea for every condition, and they're not without risks or obstacles. I've mentioned that some clinics in the US and other countries are guilty of bad science and greed—not a good combination for patients. Infection and rejection are possible, especially when clinics don't practice good hygiene and related sterile techniques.

There's also no guarantee that using exactly the right stem cells with the best techniques will work. We still have more to learn about stem and Muse cells.

- What is the optimum number of cells that need to be infused for a given condition?
- How often should the treatments be repeated (frequency) and at what dosage?
- What are the best lab techniques to help the cells replicate?
- Is it better to use the patient's own stem cells or those from another person?

That last point has been the subject of a great deal of discussion and debate. The FDA has maintained that using one's own cells involves "manipulating one's own tissues," causing the resulting product to be classified as a drug. The FDA is more tolerant of injecting donor stem cells, even though the risk, albeit low, is by nature higher than for transmitting a donor's undetected disease.

It's going to take time and research before we establish rational policies for stem cell use. The FDA categorizes mesenchymal stem cells derived from fat as an IND. Essentially, this categorization prevents doctors and other scientists from administering stem cell treatment directly to patients and gives the FDA greater regulatory control. In addition, one must submit one's stem cell study/ trial for approval by the Institutional Review Board (IRB) of one's institution, an administrative body that assesses a proposed study for safety issues. Once one files for an IND and receives approval from the IRB, one can proceed.

You should also consider "getting ahead" and prepare for future regenerative medicine treatments by banking your cells now while you're healthy, or if you believe that you may be susceptible to serious disease or chronic conditions. As mentioned, banking your cells now would allow you to lock in your current biological age and more easily access FDA expanded-use programs (right to try and compassionate use) and prepare you for immediate therapy upon FDA approval. As we age, our stem cells are also aging; "today is the youngest our cells will ever be;" I have worked extensively with American CryoStem Corporation on their medical advisory board and also serve as an investigator for their current post-concussion syndrome (PCS; also known as chronic concussive syndrome, CCS) study, "ATCELL™ Expanded Autologous, Adipose-Derived Mesenchymal Stem Cells Deployed via Intravenous Infusion for the Treatment of Post-concussion Syndrome (PCS) in Retired Military and Athletes."

This FDA-approved phase I clinical study uses regenerative cells from adipose tissue collected by liposuction to treat athletes and retired military veterans with autologous adipose-derived stem cells. To support their FDA clinical studies, and ultimately provide treatments to patients, they have created a complete platform to support adipose tissue collection, processing, cell expansion, and storage and are currently making it available to the public as a "Wellness Application" in preparation for on-demand delivery in the United States under FDA approvals and expanded access programs. All processed samples are also available to be shipped anywhere in the world on twenty-four hours' notice.

Despite some of these aforementioned obstacles, we're making rapid progress, and every day people are healing more and hurting less because of stem cells. You may need to do some legwork to find the right study or trial for you, and you may need to travel and invest financially in your treatment. But things are going to get better. While insurance doesn't cover most stem cell therapies today, this situation is bound to change. It's analogous to how insurance companies refused to cover platelet-rich plasma treatments for years, and now many do.

While primary care physicians are not the gateway to stem cell treatment at the moment, sports medicine doctors, regenerative medicine specialists, anti-aging physicians, and neurologists are becoming more active in directing their patients to stem cell therapy. Look for one of these specialists in your area if you want to enlist a medical professional in helping you access stem cells for your condition.

Best of all, Muse cell treatments are bound to advance quickly because their promise is unlimited. Once more successful trials and studies are completed and publicized, we're likely to see Muse cell therapy become the standard of care for a wide variety of conditions. For now, use your search engine to learn if a stem cell therapy trial is starting at a clinic near you.

While we are waiting for stem and Muse cell treatment to become more widely available, one treatment of note is platelet-rich plasma therapy (PRPT). PRPT is currently legal and accepted within the medical community as within proper standard of care. It is another tool for regeneration and repair that is used for conditions ranging from musculoskeletal and joint injuries to cosmetic purposes such as head hair growth and skin rejuvenation. PRPT is derived from one's own blood and essentially concentrates one's healing capabilities, to be delivered to a particular preferred area. Blood is drawn from a vein, typically at the cubital crease (front of the elbow), and the desired components are concentrated by centrifuging. Then, this concentrated result, rich in plasma and growth factors (certain hormones and bioproteins), is placed where needed.

PRPT can be used for many applications in which it makes sense to concentrate one's own healing capability and direct it where needed: a partially torn ligament or muscle, an arthritic joint, on the scalp, and even the genitals to promote healing, growth of appropriate tissue, and better function. One drawback to PRPT is that it has no value when used intravenously (we would simply be taking the platelets and growth factors out and putting them back into the blood supply), and therefore is limited to localized treatments. And, as opposed to stem cell treatments, the growth factors are there, but stem cells aren't, nor are there concentrations of typically younger, more diverse, and concentrated growth factors and messenger proteins that accompany stem cell treatments. But the potential for adverse reactions to allogeneic stem cell treatment, or other treatment such as a cortisone injection, is minimized because with PRPT one is using one's own tissue (blood).

PRPT for injuries (not cosmetic procedures) is often covered by medical insurance, but otherwise ranges in price from $1,200 to $2,000 per treatment.

9

Body Restoration Using Whole-Body Cold and Heat Therapy

MOST PEOPLE HAVE experienced the benefits of placing an ice pack or a heating pad on an aching body part. We've seen how professional athletes often take ice baths after strenuous practices or games to reduce inflammation and hardy people in cold climates plunge into freezing lakes, claiming that the experience is "invigorating." We're also aware that when we go to health clubs, people sit in extremely hot saunas, sometimes dumping buckets of cold water over their heads; they emerge feeling refreshed and as if they've sweated out the "bad stuff" in their bodies.

The value of subjecting yourself to intense cold or heat isn't just anecdotal. Research documents a variety of such physiological events that provide healthspan advantages—research that I'll share in this chapter.

Let's focus on cryotherapy first: how it works, the different ways it's administered, and the value for a wide range of conditions.

WHAT HAPPENS TO THE BODY AT 150 DEGREES BELOW ZERO

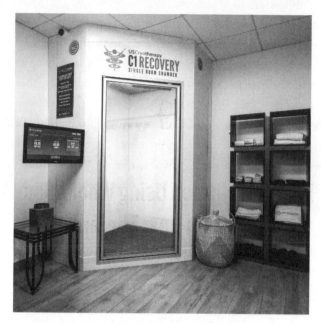

Our Electric Whole Body Cryotherapy Machine (U.S. Cryotherapy)

If you've ever seen a cryotherapy machine, you probably thought it looked like a combination high-tech refrigerator and shower. These machines vary a bit—some use nitrogen, while others produce their chill without it—but they are vertical chambers that encase you in extremely cold temperatures. While most people encounter these machines in doctors' offices or other health-related facilities, they are also available for home purchase, though they're quite expensive (low six figures).

They provide whole-body therapy and can offer multiple healthspan benefits versus treating one specific ailment. You step almost naked into the cryo chamber and the temperature goes down to somewhere between –110°F and –200°F. You're only in the chamber for a few minutes, but that's enough (over repeated treatments) to produce positive results.

Hormesis, the term that helps explain how cryotherapy works, describes the adaptive response of cells and organisms to an intermittent stressor. Think about how pearls are formed in oysters. A bit of sand enters the shell and it is just irritating enough for the oyster to form a pearl around it. When we work out, we "irritate" our muscles. We stress them just enough that the muscles become stronger and hormones are produced. Autophagy, the process of cell cleansing and repair that I described in previous chapters, works similarly; a low-dose injection of poly-phenols triggers the autophagy process.

In similar ways, spending a few minutes in a cryotherapy chamber catalyzes a variety of positive effects. Nerves that are activated by cryotherapy increase their production of cryoprotective and restorative proteins including growth factors, phase II liver detoxification, and antioxidant enzymes. Cryotherapy decreases production of cortisol, the stress hormone, as well as Dehydroepiandrosterone (DHEA), another adrenal hormone. It also decreases production of estradiol, a steroid hormone that is the most common estrogen; excessive levels of certain estrogens (estrones) can produce prostate cancer in men and cause moodiness and water retention in both men and women. Another benefit of cryotherapy: reduction of apolipoprotein B, a protein that permits LDL cholesterol to attach to cell receptors in the blood, which can help slow, stop, or even reverse CAD.

As an important aside, LDL cholesterol is not inherently bad, as so many physicians state. The sources of LDL cholesterol formation, including saturated fat, can be quite beneficial for sleep and muscle growth, just to name two examples. Just as gasoline has many beneficial uses, so, too, does LDL cholesterol. However, like gasoline stored in a five-gallon can next to a workbench where one is using an acetylene torch, LDL cholesterol in the presence of CAD is an explosion waiting to happen. Although it can fuel extant CAD, it doesn't start the process of inflammation required for plaque formation any more than gasoline by itself starts a fire.

Physiologically, the cold in cryotherapy induces vasoconstriction, the narrowing of blood vessels. After several minutes, the body reacts to compensate for the cold and induces vasodilation, the widening of the blood vessels. You see this when you go outside on a cold winter day and your cheeks become rosy. In cryotherapy, though, you go from a few minutes of cold to warmth upon leaving the chamber. The benefit of narrowing then dilating one's blood vessels is that it creates a changeover in the blood: when the blood vessels open back up, blood flow increases, which washes away bad elements in the blood such as cytokines and fosters production of restorative proteins. Cryotherapy also increases production of white blood cells.

Furthermore, intense cold stimulates dermal thermal connections. This is a fancy way of saying that the cold slows nerve conduction, creating an analgesic effect. That's why cryotherapy is so useful in treating conditions such as rheumatoid arthritis and fibromyalgia.

In addition, it catalyzes production of brown fat—the "good" or more vascularized fat that helps burn calories.

Last, cryotherapy also stimulates the release of norepinephrine, a hormone and neurotransmitter that releases energy and produces a feeling of well-being. If you've ever skied all day and then sat by the fire afterward, you've experienced that paradoxical sense of being energized but relaxed. In short, it's a terrific feeling.

THE CONDITIONS THAT IMPROVE WITH WHOLE-BODY COLD THERAPY

I've already mentioned that cryotherapy is an effective treatment for pain, making it useful for people with rheumatoid arthritis and fibromyalgia as well as ankylosing spondylitis, a form of arthritis that affects the spine. It's also useful for reducing inflammation and relieving pain from muscle strains ("pulls") and other injuries. Beyond these obvious uses, let's consider some other ways that cryotherapy benefits people:

- *Immune system.* By getting rid of cytokines and increasing the white blood cell count, cryotherapy helps our bodies fight off diseases more effectively.
- *Weight loss.* When you're cold, your body tries to stay warm by shivering; this is called thermogenesis, and by shivering you are burning calories. Regular exposure to cold creates brown fat, which burns calories. Unlike white fat, which just hangs off your body, brown fat is an energy powerhouse that produces heat to maintain your body's temperature in cold conditions.
- *Mood elevation.* Exposure to intense cold helps us feel both relaxed and energized. Some research shows that whole-body cryotherapy stimulates the release of beneficial hormones that can alleviate depression.[22]
- *Nerve-related disorders.* Research suggests that cryotherapy can help people suffering from migraines as well as pinched nerves.[23]
- *Alzheimer's disease and other neurodegenerative disorders.* Though a lot more research is needed in this area, the theory is that cryotherapy's ability to decrease inflammation and increase antioxidants may help fight the inflammation and oxidation that occurs with Alzheimer's.
- *Longevity.* By reducing free radicals, increasing cellular respiration and thermogenesis, and having other beneficial effects previously discussed, whole-body cryotherapy can contribute to helping us live longer and healthier.

OPTIONS FOR USING CRYOTHERAPY

Whole-body cryotherapy can bring benefits after only a few treatments. Many people will start out with two or three treatments of a few minutes' duration each for a week; the duration of treatment depends on their health objectives. Consider, though, that I've seen significant improvements in pain management with as little as seven total minutes weekly and these benefits can last for three months or even longer.

There's a lot of upside and little downside (aside from cost) in whole-body cryotherapy. As long as you recognize that more isn't better—you need to limit your exposure to extreme cold to no more than five minutes per session, usually less—you probably won't suffer any significant negative effects.

Still, there are some cautions. Too much cold exposure can cause cryoglobulinemia, a disorder in which blood proteins huddle together and may cause organ damage. People suffering from Raynaud's syndrome, in which blood vessels narrow in response to cold or stress, may also want to avoid cryotherapy. Because intense cold can slow down the thyroid, people with hypothyroidism likewise should probably avoid this treatment. If you have other diseases or conditions, from severe cardiovascular disease to acute respiratory system disorders, then caution may be advised. However, as with the warnings for every type of medication or treatment, these are issued not because cryotherapy is dangerous for many, but because it's dangerous for a relative few.

If you're considering whole-body therapy, the one essential precaution you should take is covering certain body parts, especially if you have a condition that makes them sensitive to extreme cold. I wear booties when I go into the cryotherapy chamber because my cervical spine injury makes my feet feel vulnerable. Many people cover their genital region, nose, mouth, and ears with some form of protection. Some people also wear head coverings in cryo chambers. Nitrogen-based cryotherapy machines are colder than electric ones, making protection even more essential; the jets on nitrogen machines shoot cold air into the chamber, which can burn one's legs if they're too close to the jets. I recommend using the electric cryotherapy chambers—I considered and selected US Cryotherapy for our cryotherapy chamber at RSM—over nitrogen for safety reasons and because the lower temperatures that nitrogen chambers can produce are not necessary.

There are also "hacks" for people who don't want to spend the money required for whole-body cryo or want a simpler, more accessible method. For instance, I bought an icemaker and ice bags and put them in the bathtub to take advantage of cold therapy at home. I also jump into our unheated pool in the winter. Neither the tub nor the pool is as cold as a cryotherapy chamber; the ice bath is around 32°F, the pool around 42°F. Nonetheless, I benefit from my parasympathetic nervous system (the portion of the autonomic nervous system responsible for repair and regeneration) kicking into action and creating that relaxed but focused feeling. It also facilitates recovery from a hard workout.

Again, you don't want to overdo these home cryo techniques. Because an ice bath is warmer than a full-body cryotherapy chamber, you can stay immersed longer—but not too long! Fifteen or twenty minutes should be the maximum time, and even "just" minutes is enough. Beyond that point, your periphery can start stealing heat from your core and you might be vulnerable to heart arrhythmias. Of course, people with atrial fibrillation, or any other heart condition, should check with their physician prior to performing cold therapy at home.

Also, if you're an athlete and just completed a workout, you should wait an hour before using cryotherapy—your body experiences beneficial inflammation after a workout, and if you do cryo too soon after exercise, you won't give your body time to provide this adaptive effect.

THE CONDITIONS THAT IMPROVE WITH WHOLE-BODY HOT THERAPY

Formally known as acute whole-body thermal therapy, this method shares certain traits and benefits with cryotherapy. Most obviously, it involves stepping into a chamber or room of extreme dry or wet heat for a limited period (to avoid overexposure). Saunas and other such enclosures are heated in various ways. Wood-burning saunas are low in humidity but higher in temperature (160°–212°F). Infrared saunas, on the other hand, use special lamps that heat the body rather than the room, the theory being that the heat/energy from infrared rays, which reaches a maximum of 140°F, penetrates farther into the body than heat from a traditional sauna, facilitating sweating in a more comfortable (i.e., less hot) environment. Steam heat (versus dry heat) is also an option and the percentage of humidity can be adjusted in some saunas.

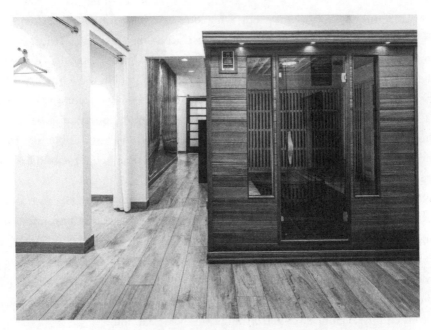

Our Infrared "Malibu" Sauna (Coastal Saunas)

All these types of heat induce metabolic changes such as heat-shock protein release. These proteins are referred to as "chaperones," in that they search for other damaged proteins that can impair cell function and escort them away from where they can do harm. The heat produces a small amount of stress in the body, catalyzing the release of these heat-shock proteins; this is part of the hormesis process that I've referred to earlier. Heat also releases beta endorphins and interleukin 6, which produce an anti-inflammatory effect. Sweating allows us to rid the body of toxins such as excess heavy metals; while we need very small amounts of heavy metals as micronutrients, too many or too much causes problems.

Heat also makes nitric oxide more available to the body, which brings a multitude of benefits and can increase insulin sensitivity, which can help with weight issues.

Now, let's translate these physiological changes to healthspan benefits. Specifically, here are some of the ways that spending time in the sauna helps us:

- ***Cardiovascular.*** Heat expands blood vessels and diminishes their stiffness, improving circulation and decreasing blood pressure. The Mayo Clinic states that saunas may have a beneficial effect on cardiovascular disease.

- *Dementia (and other neurodegenerative disorders).* Research shows that heat therapy can reduce the chances of developing neurodegenerative disorders, perhaps by increasing blood flow.
- *Breathing disorders (bronchitis, asthma, etc.).* The heat from saunas can help relax breathing muscles.
- *Sleep.* Research shows that spending a little time in a sauna and then getting into a cool bed facilitates a good night's sleep.
- *Rheumatological disorders.* Combining the anti-inflammatory and muscle-relaxing effects helps people with rheumatoid arthritis, lupus, and other chronic pain sources. Infrared saunas seem particularly useful for these types of disorders.

Saunas also seem to have a more generalized positive effect on healthspan. Dr. Jari A. Laukkanen of the University of Eastern Finland—a country that leads the world in sauna use—conducted a study in 2015 that contrasted results from infrequent (once a week) sauna use to frequent (often daily) use. For those who used the sauna more frequently, mortality rates dropped significantly, as did the risk of stroke, heart attacks, and Alzheimer's disease. Interestingly, sauna treatment can mimic cardiovascular exercise with heart rates in Zone 2 or below, which may contribute to its benefits.[24]

NAVIGATING COLD AND HOT THERAPY

As with cryotherapy, heat therapy is relatively safe for most people. Still, every treatment has a potential downside. Coronary patients can have problems with intense heat, and they should speak with their doctors before trying saunas. People with low blood pressure need to be cautious because sauna use can drop their pressure further and make them vulnerable to arrhythmias. Though this probably is obvious, going into a sauna while drinking alcohol (or drinking immediately after emerging from one) is a bad idea because the heat causes dehydration. In fact, most people should drink up to four glasses of water to replace what's lost during a typical sauna treatment. Finally, and most obviously, people who are sick or pregnant shouldn't use saunas.

In terms of how to use saunas to maximize health benefits, the common recommendation is twice-weekly sessions of no more than fifteen or twenty minutes. The type of sauna you choose is a matter of personal preference, though infrared saunas can penetrate deeper into the skin. While most people will take advantage of saunas at their health clubs, the cost of home saunas isn't as high as you might think. Infrared saunas, in particular, are advertised online for as little as $1,400.

Last, though people have been using saunas and touting the benefits of cold showers and ice baths for quite a while, relatively little research has been done on the benefits from a healthspan perspective. It's entirely possible that researchers will find other benefits beyond the ones that I've noted, as well as better ways to use cold and heat therapeutically. For instance, we've learned that alternating hot and cold can amplify the effect on health; going from a sauna to an ice bath can have a synergistic rather than just an additive impact.

In the future, we will discover other ways to mix and fine-tune these whole-body therapies and improve their effects. Until then, heat and cold provide affordable, accessible options for everyone to improve their healthspan.

10

Staying Younger with Hyperbaric Oxygen Therapy

IF YOU'VE EVER watched any documentaries or other shows about deep-sea diving, you probably are aware of a disorder called "the bends," more formally known as decompression sickness. It describes what happens when divers surface too quickly and develop nitrogen bubbles in their blood and tissues from the decrease in pressure. These bubbles can create all sorts of problems, from headaches to death.

To treat this problem, divers are placed in hyperbaric oxygen chambers, pressurized environments that provide 100 percent oxygen either through vents or, more commonly, masks. This changes the nitrogen into more easily absorbed liquid form and usually helps divers eliminate their symptoms or reduce the damage.

Though you may not be a deep-sea diver, you can still derive significant healthspan benefits from hyperbaric oxygen therapy (HBOT).

HOW HYPERBARIC OXYGEN WORKS

There are two types of HBOT chambers, hard and soft. The latter are smaller with soft walls and may be portable; they can only be pressurized to a lesser degree and are considerably cheaper ($20,000). The former have hard walls and are larger; they can be pressurized higher and are very expensive ($250,000 and up). Both can be effective, depending on the patient's disorder and treatment objective.

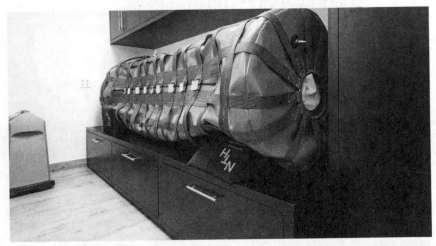

Our Soft Monoplace Hyperbaric Oxygen Chamber (Newtowne Hyperbarics)

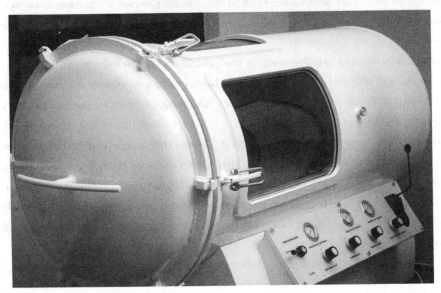

Hard Monoplace Hyperbaric Oxygen Chamber

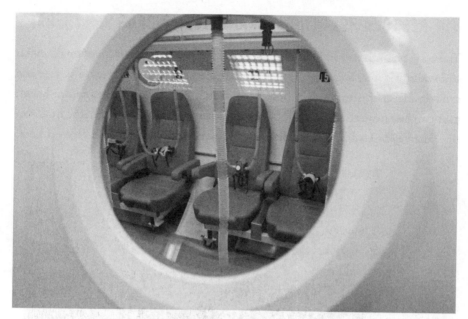

Hard Multiplace Oxygen Chamber

There are also two subtypes by capacity: monoplace (usually for one person) and multiplace (for six or more).

HBOT delivers oxygen in a pressurized environment. Typically, the oxygen is delivered through masks rather than vents that fill the entire chamber with oxygen. The latter can be dangerous—a single spark can create a massive explosion and fire.

The pressurized environment is the critical factor, though, because it drives oxygen deeper into the body. Think of it this way: the oxygen in the air at sea level is about 20 percent or 0.2 atmospheres. Switching to 100 percent oxygen, or 1 atmosphere, represents a huge increase.

The atmospheric pressure is often 2.5 times that at sea level in hard chambers and 1.5 times in soft chambers. This higher pressure compresses the oxygen and allows it to travel into smaller vessels at higher concentrations. In short, it brings more oxygen to more parts of your body than you would ordinarily receive. Once your hemoglobin is saturated, the oxygen is pushed into the blood and then the tissues.

Now let's examine the many different ways this pressurized oxygen helps us.

THE RESTORATIVE BENEFITS OF HYPERBARIC OXYGEN THERAPY

You may be surprised to learn that HBOT has a wide range of benefits, far wider than conditions related to its original purpose of treating divers who surface too quickly. It's unsurprising, however, that there's some disagreement among various agencies about what conditions and disorders are best served by HBOT.

The FDA lists fourteen different approved health issues for HBOT treatment:

- Air or gas embolism
- Carbon monoxide poisoning
- Healing diabetes-caused wounds
- Crush injuries
- Decompression sickness
- Arterial injuries
- Necrotizing soft tissue infections
- Severe anemia
- Intracranial abscesses
- Osteomyelitis
- Delayed radiation injury
- Compromised skin grafts
- Thermal skin injuries
- Idiopathic (disease of unknown origin) hearing loss

The Mayo Clinic has its own list of approved treatments, which include traumatic brain injury, vision loss, and radiation injuries.

I've seen a lot of convincing research that HBOT also helps people with Bell's palsy, asthma, depression, certain migraine types, hepatitis, Parkinson's disease, Alzheimer's disease, and spinal cord injuries, and can act as adjunct therapy for HIV. Personally, I've found that HBOT facilitates recovery after intense bike riding excursions with professional riders; it helps me feel as good on the fourth day of climbing as on the first. Other serious athletes swear that it also helps them recover from intense workouts.

Though not FDA approved for the following, some evidence exists that HBOT is a useful treatment for people who have suffered strokes, have traumatic brain injuries, and for post-traumatic stress disorder. It's also a good technique for releasing stem cells from bone marrow as well as helping create stem cells, which we know has a myriad of benefits.[25]

HBOT may have value as a complementary cancer treatment. Let's take a moment to explain how this is possible. Cancer cells create their own blood supplies by forming a system of aberrant blood vessels. These new blood vessels are not particularly well formed, having originated in a hypoxic or low-oxygen environment. The theory is that when we compress oxygen, we increase the concentration of oxygen that reaches cancer cells. The pressure produced in HBOT results in hyperoxidation, which kills the cancer cells, especially when combined with a 10-gram or higher (pro-oxidative) dose of vitamin C.

In addition, HBOT may be able to increase the effectiveness of radiation therapy. Radiation kills cancer cells through reactive oxygen species, which is toxic to cancer, and the use of HBOT just prior to this treatment may increase the number of cancer cells killed. HBOT sensitizes the microenvironment to respond to radiation by forcing oxygen into tumor tissue that is otherwise hypoxic (devoid of oxygen). Healthy tissue becomes much more resistant to the inflammatory effects of radiation.

Just as important, because HBOT helps release and create stem cells, it may have value as a preventive cancer tactic by mobilizing stem cells to home in on cells that need repair before they grow out of control. It's important to note that in both human and animal studies, HBOT alone has never been found to increase survivorship for any type of cancer. Future studies and improved HBOT best practices may reveal ways to use HBOT to improve survival rates. For now, though, it remains a promising complementary therapy.

DECIDING IF HYPERBARIC OXYGEN THERAPY IS FOR YOU

If you're considering HBOT, be aware that though it's generally safe for most people, some cautions exist.

First, make sure someone is monitoring you while you're in the chamber. Though seizures are rare, pressurized pure oxygen can cause them, especially if you've had a traumatic brain injury. If you're receiving oxygen through an actual mask versus through a vent in an acrylic chamber, someone should be ready to intervene in the event of a seizure and remove the mask, which will prevent serious harm in most instances.

Second, middle-ear trauma is possible if you fail to clear your ears when in the chamber. The Valsalva maneuver is a technique that allows you to reverse the imbalance of pressure in your ears by pinching your nose closed, closing your mouth, and compressing air out of your lungs into the ear canals for about five seconds. You should also use the Valsalva maneuver if your ears clog while in the chamber. The trick is to use the maneuver *before* your ears begin to feel too much pressure buildup, which makes the pressure imbalance easier to reverse.

Third, if you're prone to claustrophobia, a small chamber may not be for you.

Fourth, a small but significant risk to the lens of the eye exists. Specifically, some people receiving HBOT have reported myopic vision changes and the creation and exacerbation of cataracts.

Fifth, it may require an investment of time. If you're using HBOT for treatment of carbon monoxide poisoning, you probably only need a few treatments. If you're treating certain diseases or something like a nonhealing diabetic wound, you may require thirty or more treatments for thirty days in a row (or sixty days if you do it every other day). Given that a single treatment is usually an hour, but can range from a few minutes to two hours or more, HBOT can require a significant commitment.

In terms of cost, most people don't buy their own HBOT chambers. As mentioned, the soft-shell models cost around $20,000 while the larger, hard-shell models can be $250,000 or more. Many communities do have HBOT facilities, though. If you're being treated for an FDA-approved condition, insurance will probably cover it. If it's not FDA approved, the hard chamber may cost around $250 per session and the soft chamber perhaps $100 per session.

Last, I should point out that HBOT is terrific for general healthspan purposes in addition to treating specific conditions. Treatment stimulates an immune response that may raise the levels of glutathione, a powerful antioxidant, and the enzyme superoxide dismutase. Both of these substances break down when we age. If we can raise their levels through HBOT, they'll help rid our bodies of free radicals, which catalyze various diseases. Plus, the more glutathione we have, the better able it is to recharge our vitamin C. Together, they form a potent weapon against cell damage.

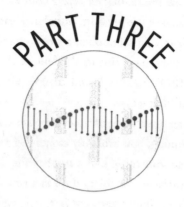

PART THREE

Four Anti-aging Tools for Leveling the Longevity Playing Field

Metformin for Mitigating Diabetes and Other Premature Aging Conditions

IN THE 1940S, scientists developed a glucose-lowering drug from the French lilac. Over the years, this drug evolved into the one now known as metformin, a prescription drug for diabetes. While the mechanism by which metformin works isn't completely understood, it decreases glucose production in the liver by about one-third and also reduces absorption of glucose from the intestines. The most common side effects are gastrointestinal problems in about one in five patients. It also inhibits how vitamin B12 is absorbed, though patients can take supplements to counteract this effect. Furthermore, metformin can contribute to a rare condition called lactic acidosis, an excessive buildup of lactic acid, so patients with type 2 diabetes who also suffer from impaired kidney function usually receive lower-than-normal doses of metformin. Other than these issues, this is a time-tested, safe, and inexpensive drug.

As good as metformin is in treating type 2 diabetes, its potential ability to improve healthspan is even more exciting. In a 2014 study published in a British pharmacological journal, the authors reported an astonishing discovery: study subjects with diabetes being treated with metformin lived longer than "healthier" control subjects (people who didn't have diabetes).[26] Logically, people suffering from diabetes (or any major disease) would probably not live as long as people who didn't have the disease. That metformin reversed this logic by increasing longevity was significant.

We don't understand everything about how metformin works to protect us from the diseases of aging, but we have some important clues. You'll recall our discussion of mitochondria as the powerhouses of the cell. Metformin essentially works on mitochondria to inhibit the production of energy. In doing so, it fosters the illusion that the cell is being starved. In addition to making adenosine triphosphate (ATP), the primary source of energy that facilitates muscular

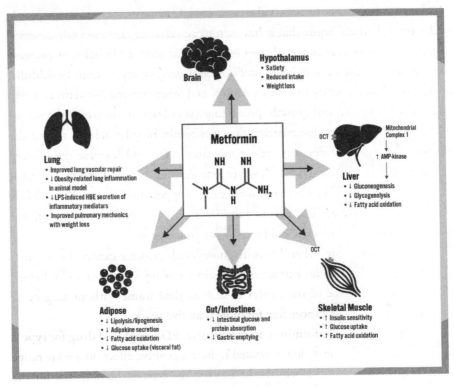

Metformin's Multiple and Various Effects

contraction, cellular production of adenosine-monophosphate-activated protein kinase (AMPK), a protein with enzymatic function, is upregulated when we exercise. AMPK improves insulin sensitivity on cell surfaces and thereby improves transport of sugars into cells. It also stops production of fatty acids and blocks absorption of sugar from the intestines, helping fight obesity. By decreasing oxidative stress and inflammation, it also may prevent Alzheimer's and heart disease. In the facing graphic, LPS stands for lipopolysaccharides; their reduction can be important in that they are pro-inflammatory. In this example, the reference is to LPS-induced inflammation of HBE (human bronchial epithelial) cells, and how the use of metformin reduces this inflammation. The reference to OCT (organic cation transporter) simply shows the mechanism by which metformin is affecting the liver and skeletal muscle.

METFORMIN AND MINIMIZING THE SPREAD OF CANCER CELLS

Metformin also seems to have value as a complementary treatment for people with cancer; I would argue that it has even more value for treating early-detected cancers. We know that cancer thrives on sugar and metformin helps us decrease the amount of glucose our body produces and process sugar more healthfully. More than that, its ability to activate AMPK and other enzymes/proteins can stop protein synthesis and cell growth, preventing (or at least minimizing) the spread of cancer cells. Studies demonstrate that metformin may be able to reduce the number of cancers we develop, reduce mortality rates, and increase the efficacy of radiation and chemotherapy. However, one significant caveat shown in recent research is that, while not the norm, some cancers appear to do better with AMPK activation. So, as always, it is best to consider the use of metformin as an adjunct to cancer treatment under the guidance of your oncologist.[27]

On a personal note, when I was diagnosed with prostate cancer, I took metformin along with green tea extract as the mainstay of my treatment and it helped me eliminate any trace of the cancer in a short time frame without surgery or irradiation. I have been cancer free for more than five years.

All this is to say: metformin is an inexpensive, FDA-approved drug for type 2 diabetes that has also been demonstrated to have a positive effect on a wide range of diseases when used off-label. The best news, however, is the potential for the drug to help us live longer and better.

THE TAME STUDY

Dr. Nir Barzilai, an endocrinologist and director of the Institute for Aging Research at the Albert Einstein College of Medicine, is in the process of conducting a possibly groundbreaking study on aging: Targeting Aging with Metformin (TAME). The possible results may be groundbreaking, not just because of the study's goal—demonstrating that metformin can delay the onset of aging-related conditions such as Alzheimer's, heart disease, and cancer—but, if successful, the TAME study can open the door to classifying aging as a disease. When this happens, we're going to see much greater interest in and production of anti-aging drugs and other treatments. Because this is a high-profile, randomized, double-blind, placebo-controlled study, it has the capacity to generate a great deal of publicity as well as pressure on the FDA to approve effective products.

A number of other concurrent studies on metformin and aging may also help legitimize anti-aging medicine. These studies include a major one being conducted by the Department of Veterans Affairs with almost eight thousand enrolled adults that's focusing on metformin's effect on prediabetes patients and subsequent heart disease, as well as one being conducted by the University of Texas Health Science Center, sponsored by the National Institute on Aging, examining how metformin might affect frailty in older adults.

One of the aging theories I mentioned earlier is DNA methylation—how it affects our biological versus chronological age. Recent studies demonstrate that metformin positively affects DNA methylation both globally (genome wide) and locally (within each organ). Increasingly, everyone from scientists to laypersons are interested in how this theory helps them assess their real age. If we can figure out what causes undesirable DNA methylation, we might be able to slow the aging process. The idea of being sixty chronologically, but only forty biologically has a powerful hold on our imaginations. If more people become aware of the notion of one's real age, it's going to spur greater interest in anti-aging medicine.

All of this is critical for people who want to take advantage of metformin. Even though it's FDA-approved for type 2 diabetes, some doctors won't approve of it for anything except treating that disease. Despite establishment medicine's reluctance to prescribe metformin to enhance cellular function and as a preventive medicine approach to anti-aging, we're seeing a growing demand for it to be approved for off-label use.

My experience is that the gastrointestinal side effects tend to appear more often in people taking metformin for diabetes than those taking it for anti-aging or preventive purposes.

ALTERNATIVES TO METFORMIN: GYNOSTEMMA AND BERBERINE

If you are one of the relatively small number of people who are unable to tolerate metformin at any dosage or can't obtain a prescription, consider two over-the-counter alternatives that appear to work the same or similarly to metformin by lowering blood sugar, activating AMPK, and agonizing peroxisome-proliferator-activated receptors (PPAR) that, when some types are activated, lower blood sugar and triglycerides and help treat metabolic syndromes like diabetes. These alternatives are gynostemma and berberine.

Gynostemma is derived from an herb also used in Chinese medicine, and has been used to treat diabetes as well as other conditions. Berberine has been compared favorably with metformin in various studies and can be taken in the same dosage, milligram for milligram, as that drug. It doesn't produce the same gastrointestinal difficulties as metformin, but it's more expensive.

Whichever substance you decide to take, the work of Dr. Nir Barzilai and others suggest that it is never too late to start and that taking some is better than taking none. While a maximum recommended dose exists for each—the recommended daily dosage for metformin, for example, is 2,550 mg in divided doses or 2,000 mg daily in its extended-release form—an advantage to taking these medications is that you cannot lower blood glucose too far with them. One of the risks when using many of the other diabetes drugs for lowering blood sugar (such as insulin) is that blood sugar can be decreased too far, even to a deadly level. Not so with the maximum daily dosage of metformin, berberine, or gynostemma.

HOW TO TEST IF METFORMIN IS RIGHT FOR YOUR LONGEVITY PLAN

Thankfully and remarkably, given that close to one-third of all Americans are living with pre-diabetes or type 2 diabetes, one can obtain metformin for less than $10 a month.[28]

If you are interested in using metformin as an anti-aging approach or to prevent one of the diseases we've discussed, then you can request that your regular physician prescribe it to you "off-label" for something other than the condition that it's FDA approved to treat. Some doctors are willing to do this, but others aren't. You might consider showing your doctor the studies referenced in this chapter—there is a lot of solid science attesting to metformin's value as an anti-aging medication—and all this research might be sufficient to catalyze a prescription. If not, you may have to see a more sympathetic doctor (an anti-aging medicine specialist, for instance) to obtain a prescription.

To avoid or minimize the drug's gastrointestinal side effects, you can build up your dosage slowly, take it with food, and use an extended-release metformin capsule so that instead of getting one large dose all at once, you spread out the effects of the medication. Typically, when I prescribe metformin for patients, I have them take one capsule at dinner and monitor how they do for a week. If they tolerate it well, I increase it to one capsule at dinner and one at breakfast. Capsules are usually between 250 mg and 500 mg and I slowly increase the daily dose as tolerated to its maximum.

12

Using Peptides to Prolong Life

IF YOU'VE EVER been a bodybuilder or other type of athlete, you may have taken a peptide, a molecular chain of two or more amino acids. It may have been creatine, a peptide that helps build muscle and aid recovery from exercise. Or, if you're concerned about your skin's appearance, you may use a lotion with peptides that create or maintain collagen.

Peptides adapted for medical use aren't new; approximately 10 percent of pharmaceuticals are peptide and protein based. What's new, however, is the growing recognition that peptides possess a wide range of therapeutic properties.

Think of peptides as an almost endless series of Tinkertoy designs, where numerous possibilities exist for how they're built. Each possibility is linked to different healthcare goals. A peptide is similar to a protein but smaller; it's a molecule of between two and fifty amino acids (proteins contain more than fifty amino acids), strung together in many different combinations. Peptides occur naturally in many foods, but we've learned that we can increase their effectiveness by creating synthetic peptides.

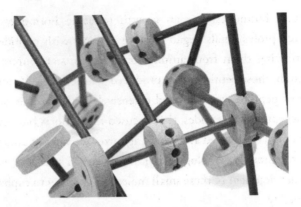

Tinkertoys © Can Stock Photo / kozzi

Peptides are so effective therapeutically because cell membranes possess many channels and receptors involved in biochemical reactions that depend on peptides. We therefore can use peptides—primarily through injections but also in pills, inhaled sprays, and lotions—to catalyze the reaction we want. Not only can peptides stimulate the body to produce more or less of a substance like hormones—for instance, producing more growth hormone—but they can also be used to enhance normal functions and treat dysfunctions.

To communicate the potential of peptides for a wide variety of conditions, let me share my own eye-opening experience when I first learned about peptides.

PEPTIDES: THE LONGEVITY BUILDING BLOCKS

During pre-med, I was walking to a class in the physics building and on the building's walls were drawings of peptides. Their intricate structures were compelling viewing, a kind of art. I asked a professor why these pictures were displayed in the physics building, given that they were more appropriate for the biology wing of the school. The teacher explained that physics is all about structure and that was why they were exhibited in this particular building.

As I looked at these structures, I was struck by the vast therapeutic value of peptides. Even when I was just a student, it was apparent that we could create an infinite variety of combinations, all of which engaged the cell in different ways for different health-related goals.

The first peptides used therapeutically replaced or supplemented peptides that we produce naturally, such as insulin. Many of the body's hormones are peptides, including thyroid hormones, human growth releasing hormones, and adrenaline. Healthcare professionals began treating patients with peptides as early as the 1920s, extracting them from animals or other natural sources. Starting in the 1950s, though, most peptides were produced synthetically. Venoms, a typical animal source of peptides, were studied extensively early on, but once scientists identified the receptors for peptides, they focused their efforts on creating smaller molecules that could be injected and would agonize (activate) or antagonize (deactivate) peptide receptors. Technology, including recent AI advances, has facilitated the laboratory development of these small molecules as a way to capitalize on peptides therapeutically.

Over time, we've learned a lot about how supplementing peptides can influence healthspan. For instance, we've proved they can rebuild muscle and enhance skin appearance. But a great deal of ongoing research provides evidence of peptides' effectiveness for stopping the growth of cancer, protecting the heart, managing diabetes, and improving longevity. Because most of my patients are trying to optimize their health, as opposed to curing or managing an existing disease, I've found peptides to be particularly useful for proactively enhancing and maintaining good health, as well as speeding recovery from various injuries.

PEPTIDES AND THE IMMUNE SYSTEM

The pandemic has made people more aware of their immune systems and how exercise, sleep, and nutrition can help strengthen their disease resistance. As we age, we may experience a decline in function of the thymus gland—the Grand Central Station of the immune system. Located in the upper chest, the thymus produces immune cells. If it makes fewer of these cells as we become older, we become more vulnerable to disease. One study used a peptide combined with two other hormones to regenerate thymus tissue, restoring its efficacy as an immune system regulator. While this study needs more review, it's promising in that we know peptides can regenerate thymus tissue and help people with immune systems compromised by allergies or autoimmune diseases.

Though we obtain peptides naturally from the food we consume, this is not a particularly efficient delivery system because stomach acid breaks peptides apart before they reach the cell membrane. The size of peptide molecules is another obstacle; they are often too large to be absorbed through the intestinal membrane or sublingually. As a result, we usually inject peptides directly into the bloodstream, though certain peptides can be applied directly to the skin or via other delivery systems.

Peptides aren't perfect. Their relatively short half-life (the time it takes for a drug to be metabolized and excreted) can limit the sustained benefit of any given peptide, with the exception of sermorelin and tesamorelin (growth hormone stimulating peptides) being good examples of peptides with appropriately acute benefits. Taking too much of some peptides and creating a surplus of a desired hormone can also be problematic; many of the systems stimulated by peptides are governed by self-regulating mechanisms (negative feedback loops) that prevent creating a surplus.

Additionally, be aware that the laws relating to peptides are somewhat confusing. While the FDA has approved some peptides for specific uses, others are illegal. For instance, human growth hormone (HGH)—actually, by definition, a protein rather than a peptide since it contains a total of 191 amino acids—is illegal in this country if prescribed off-label; it is legal to prescribe it for certain conditions, like dwarfism in children. While PT-141 is an FDA-approved peptide designed to increase female libido, it isn't approved for male libido, but some doctors prescribe it off-label for this purpose. Although most pharmacies carry only FDA-approved peptides, some will sell peptides that aren't FDA approved. Underground sources exist for especially popular peptides, but the quality can vary wildly and, per the FDA, all peptides require a prescription.

Despite these negatives, many peptides provide real alternatives to traditional treatments. They are relatively safe, effective, inexpensive, and they usually don't have serious side effects. There are major exceptions to this, such as adrenaline and insulin, which can kill when taken in high enough doses, but most of the health-optimizing peptides I describe next are very safe. In Western medicine, we tend to place all of our bets on a single, powerful pill. The problem is that some of them cause powerful side effects. Ultimately, the ability of artificial intelligence to generate likely-candidate compounds, combined with further experimentation, should enable us to create combinations of peptides that are more effective than any single treatment. One pairing we're already prescribing is the peptide BPC-157 with L-glutamine to treat gastritis. This treatment has few significant, if any, side effects, especially compared to how gastritis is often treated.

HOW PEPTIDES HELP YOU HAVE MORE VITALITY

My perspective on peptides is influenced by my medical practice. I've found peptides to be extremely useful when it comes to mind and body performance improvement, body composition, sexual enhancement, and longevity. Every day seems to bring a new study about the benefits of peptides for a startlingly wide variety of diseases and disorders. Though I'm loath to temper this enthusiasm, I would raise a yellow flag and note that the claims made for peptides sometimes recall the old *Saturday Night Live* sketch for a product called "Shimmer," touted as both a "floor wax and a dessert topping."

Some things are too good to be true, so exhibiting at least some caution with regard to claims is wise. With this caveat in mind, let's examine some of the varied uses of peptides to treat different conditions.

GROWTH HORMONE PRODUCTION

Many different products and formulations exist to stimulate production of growth hormone. I've listed a number of them because there's so much interest in this hormone, especially because of references to it as the new fountain of youth. While it may not be what Ponce de León was looking for, it does seem to help people look and feel younger, particularly with its ability to increase skin thickness and turgor, reduce fat stores, and regenerate both tendons and ligaments. This latter benefit is especially important for the elderly, since a significant percentage of older people fall, break a hip, and die shortly thereafter. The theory is that if they can develop greater muscle, tendon, and ligament strength (as well as balance) using growth hormone, they might avoid this outcome, although the use of a substance such as an anabolic steroid (a cholesterol-based hormone that enhances muscle growth and strength) would more often be a better alternative to growth hormone.

I've also observed a phenomenon associated with some people who enhance their growth hormone levels; you may have seen this effect in individuals you know. You haven't seen John or Mary for months or even longer, and when you encounter them, they look fabulous. You ask them if they have been working out or following a special diet, and they respond, "No, I've simply added taking peptides that create growth hormones to my routine."

Here are some of the growth-hormone-stimulating peptide types of which you should be aware:

Ibutamoren (peptidomimetic). Also known as MK-677, ibutamoren is a peptidomimetic rather than a pure peptide, meaning it acts like a peptide but is not one in the scientific definition of the term. It's a *secretagogue*, stimulating the production of growth hormone (*secreted* by the anterior pituitary gland) to increase its levels in the body. It is also one of the best in this category and easiest to use. Most peptides need to be injected, but ibutamoren can be swallowed like any pill with a sip of water. It works via the ghrelin system (GHS-R1a, a.k.a. growth hormone secretagogue receptor 1a) and, in my experience, usually provides similar or better results than the true peptides in this category. Taking an exogenous growth hormone can create excess levels of this hormone, which may be useful for certain conditions, like surgical recovery, but can also create a number of problems including discouraging your own body from producing as much of this hormone as is normal or even producing it at all. Using a secretagogue, however, induces recrudescence (a fancy way of saying "renewal") in the area of the pituitary gland that produces growth hormone, so that one can often eventually use less secretagogue to get the same result. The risk of using too much growth hormone that accompanies exogenous growth hormone use is eliminated by using a secretagogue, which stimulates endogenous production and is therefore regulated by what is called a "negative feedback loop." Simply put, no matter how much a secretagogue is used to increase production of growth hormone, there is a maximum level of hormone recognized by the body at which any signals from a secretagogue will be ignored, causing a negative effect on production.

One minor drawback to ibutamoren and any of the secretagogues that work through the ghrelin pathway is the side effect of hunger. Like any secretagogue that uses this pathway, it creates ghrelin activation— the same source of hunger associated with marijuana use ("the munchies"). However, as with all the growth-hormone-releasing secretagogues, if you take it right before bed, you'll probably be asleep (typical sleep latency is 12 to 14 minutes) and therefore avoid this hungry feeling. Last, some patients occasionally experience initial water retention that usually reverses completely after two or three weeks.

Common dosing protocols for ibutamoren range from 12.5 mg to 25 mg, administered by mouth at bedtime, with a 30-day supply costing around $200.

Ipamorelin. This peptide works similarly to ibutamoren, but with few or no hunger side effects or the temporary water retention associated with ibutamoren. It is also injected rather than taken orally.

Common dosing protocols for ipamorelin range from 200 mcg to 300 mcg, administered once nightly via subcutaneous injection, with a 5 mg bottle (reconstituted with bacteriostatic water) costing around $180.

Sermorelin. One of the first treatments developed to treat dwarfism in an attempt to increase the body's production of growth hormone (GH), sermorelin is a short-acting peptide that works by mimicking the action of GH-releasing hormone (GHRH). Originally branded as Geref and now improved as tesamorelin with a longer half-life and increased efficacy, sermorelin is actually the first twenty-nine amino acids of the forty-six amino acid sequence that make up the actual GHRH produced by the body. Like all GH-releasing secretagogues, it should be taken nightly before bed and on a relatively empty stomach (no food two to three hours prior). Eating closer to bedtime tends to increase blood sugar and, more importantly, insulin, which tends to blunt the response to a GH secretagogue and thus counters GH production.

One disadvantage to sermorelin is that some individuals experience an allergic reaction to it. While this does not seem to affect the efficacy of the peptide, it is a nuisance (pruritus and flushing) that could discourage people from taking sermorelin appropriately. In addition, after approximately ninety days, sermorelin tends to have reduced efficacy, so you must suspend its use for a time before restarting. It also makes some people drowsy and improves sleep quality, which sometimes makes it the preferred choice among the GH secretagogues, even though others are more effective at stimulating GH release.

Common dosing protocols for sermorelin can range from 200 to 1,000 mcg, administered at bedtime via subcutaneous injection, with a 30 mg supply (reconstituted with bacteriostatic water) costing around $200.

MUSCLE GROWTH

Thymosin beta-4. This peptide helps build muscle through proliferation of actin fibers, particularly when muscle tissue has been damaged, but also provides advantages to older athletes trying to maintain their exercise regimens. It has been identified as a "moonlighting" peptide because it also regenerates tissue and reduces inflammation. Thymosin beta-4 appears to promote the migration of certain cells to an area of injury (such as heart damage after a heart attack) and the differentiation of stem cells and formation of new blood vessels. Multiple clinical trials are underway to evaluate the efficacy of thymosin beta-4 on a variety of conditions involving regeneration and inflammation including the heart, cornea, skin, gastrointestinal tract, and endothelial (inner lining of the vasculature) tissue.

Common dosing protocols for thyomosin beta-4 range from 500 mg to 1,000 mg administered daily via subcutaneous injection (reconstituted with bacteriostatic water), with a 5 mg bottle costing around $300.

Follistatin 344 & 315. You'll recall that I noted how peptides can be agonists or antagonists, promoting or reducing the body's production of a given substance. Follistatin 344 & 315 represent the latter type. Myostatin (a.k.a. growth differentiation factor 8, GDF-8) is a peptide hormone (myokine) that inhibits the growth and differentiation of muscle cells (myogenesis). By blocking the production of myostatin, we can produce and maintain muscle more easily. Myostatin inhibitors such as follistatin 344 & 315 show such promise that they are being studied as a potential therapy for muscular dystrophy, which is a group of genetically derived disorders that leads to loss and weakness of muscle tissue as well as associated organ dysfunction. They are also banned by the World Anti-Doping Agency.

Common dosing protocols for follistatin range from 50 mcg to 100 mcg daily, administered via subcutaneous injection (reconstituted with bacteriostatic water), with a 1 mg bottle costing around $175.

PEG-MGF. While this peptide is related to growth hormone, it also is a fraction (splice variant) of insulin-like growth factor–1 (IGF-1), which is more specifically related to muscle growth. MGF stands for "mechano growth factor" and induces hypertrophy (growth/repair) of damaged muscle. Because MGF has a very short half-life, we've PEGylated (added chains of polyethylene glycol polymer) the MGF structure to increase how long it works. Current research is focused on its use to repair damaged heart muscle after heart attacks, but researchers and patients are also using it to help increase or maintain muscle mass.

Common dosing protocols from PEG-MGF range from 100 mcg to 500 mcg, once daily via subcutaneous injection (reconstituted with bacteriostatic water), with a 5 mg bottle costing around $80.

TENDON AND GASTROINTESTINAL REPAIR

BPC-157. Using human gastric pentadecapeptide body protection compound (BPC), which was discovered in and isolated from human gastric juice, scientists developed a partial sequence of fifteen amino acids called pentadecapeptide BPC-157 (BPC-157 for short). It is shown to promote healing of tendons, skin, corneas, muscles, the gastrointestinal tract, and can help with erectile dysfunction because of its effect on endothelial nitric oxide synthase. It is also currently being evaluated in clinical trials for the treatment of inflammatory bowel diseases (e.g., Crohn's and ulcerative colitis).

BPC-157 is commonly used by athletes to help them recover more quickly from training and to expedite healing of acute injuries to tendons and ligaments, as well as address inflammation in joints. One can review some of the basic science in animal studies to better understand BPC-157's mechanism of action.[29] Typical human protocols will consist of site injections (via a very small 32-gauge insulin needle) in or around the area designated for treatment, at dosages of 2 mcg/kg of body weight (200–400 mcg as an average range) twice per day for four to twelve weeks. BPC-157 can also be administered systemically via subcutaneous injections.

As always, working with your physician to source pharma-grade BPC-157 and carefully monitor its effects is the place to start. At time of printing, a 5 mg bottle (which must be reconstituted with bacteriostatic water) of BPC-157 is around $350. Notably, there are also oral and nasal preparations of BPC-157. Last, you can find a good survey of the effects of BPC-157 as recorded in past animal studies.[30]

COGNITIVE ENHANCEMENT

Cerebrolysin. This is a nootropic, a broad category for any substance that may have a positive impact on mental health and cognitive function. Cerebrolysin, the brand name for porcine-brain-derived proteolytic peptide fraction (FPE 1070 or FPF 1070), has been shown to demonstrate statistically significant improvements in mental status in Alzheimer's disease patients and is used by those otherwise healthy in the belief that it may prevent Alzheimer's disease and improve cognition. It possesses both neuroprotective and neurotrophic repair properties similar to other nerve growth factors and it passes through the blood–brain barrier. Cerebrolysin is also being studied for its effectiveness in treating Parkinson's disease, multiple sclerosis, Lou Gehrig's disease (a.k.a. amyotrophic lateral sclerosis), and damage resulting from stroke and traumatic brain injury.

Common protocols for cerebrolysin can range up to 5 mL daily via intramuscular injection (reconstituted with bacteriostatic water), with 5 mg ampules costing around $200.

FGL(L). The FG loop peptide is a variant of the naturally occurring neural cell adhesion molecule with neurotrophic (nerve regenerating) and neuroprotective properties. It helps heal neurons and decrease oxidative-stress-induced neuronal cell death. It is being used to treat symptoms related to Alzheimer's disease progression and to improve memory and general cognitive function. In addition to using it for neurodegenerative disease, healthcare professionals are assessing its use for the treatment of damage and depression following stroke and traumatic brain injury.

Common dosing protocols for FGL(L) can range from 100 mg to 200 mg daily via subcutaneous injection (reconstituted with bacteriostatic water), with a 10 mg bottle costing around $550.

LIBIDO AND ERECTILE DYSFUNCTION

PT-141. This peptide, also called bremelanotide and now sold in the US under the brand name Vyleesi, emerged as a result of initial testing of another peptide, melanotan II, developed for tanning of the skin. One of the scientists involved in the early testing of melanotan II unintentionally injected himself with twice the dose and experienced an eight-hour erection accompanied by nausea and vomiting. While melanotan II eventually proved to be effective in increasing skin pigmentation, nine of the original ten test subjects (male) experienced spontaneous erections and sexual arousal. By tinkering with the composition of the melanotan II peptide, PT-141 was developed solely for the purpose of increasing both male and female libido and treating erectile dysfunction in men. The FDA has approved its use for treatment of generalized hypoactive sexual desire disorder in premenopausal women without an underlying identifiable cause, but it is also used off-label for increasing libido in both men and women with or without underlying conditions as an effective alternative to phosphodiesterase type 5 (PDE-5) enzyme inhibitors such as Viagra, Levitra, Cialis, and Stendra for male erectile dysfunction.

Common protocols for PT-141 range from 1 mg (for men) to 2 mg (for women) as needed, via subcutaneous injection (reconstituted via bacteriostatic water), with a 10 mg bottle costing around $275.

TANNING

Melanotan II. Admittedly, tanning is usually considered cosmetic, a less serious goal than those of other peptides. Still, enhancing appearance is not a superficial objective in that it can both foster a sense of well-being and confidence, as well as offer protection to fair-skinned people from damaging UV radiation. I also include it here because it demonstrates the wide range of peptide effects. This particular peptide is an analog (closely resembling in structure and similar-acting substance) of human alpha-melanocyte-stimulating hormone (alpha-MSH) that induces pigmentation (melanogenesis) in the skin. It was developed to protect fair-skinned people from sun exposure and possible skin cancer. As a nice side effect, it often creates a tanned look. A caution: melanotan II can also produce a less attractive grayish-brown skin color in fair-skinned people and those who use more than recommended doses. It also has a mild fat-loss effect and an aphrodisiac effect in men and women as well as an erectile-function effect in men. The FDA has approved melanotan I (a similar analog of melanotan II) under the brand name Scenesse in the

US to prevent skin damage from sun exposure for those with the disorder erythropoietic protoporphyria.

Common protocols for melanotan II can range from 250 mg to 500 mcg daily via subcutaneous injection (reconstituted with bacteriostatic water), with a 10 mg bottle costing around $250.

TESTOSTERONE DEFICIENCY

Kisspeptin-10. Kisspeptins are neuroendocrine peptides that stimulate the release of gonadotropin-releasing hormone, catalyzing the release of testosterone. Kisspeptins are also linked to improved egg implantation and maturation and can prevent ectopic pregnancy in women. Kisspeptins are further being studied for their link to suppression of malignant melanoma and breast cancer.

Various protocols are used with kisspeptin, and the average monthly cost is $350.

OSTEOARTHRITIS

AOD 9604. This is a modified form of amino acids 176 through 191 in the human growth hormone. As with other peptides, this compound's initial purpose changed as it was being studied. Originally, its effect on reducing fat stores was studied and, while it performed wonderfully in animal trials, it failed to meet criteria in human phase III clinical trials. However, it has shown promise as a stimulant for bone and cartilage regeneration as well as a treatment for lowering cholesterol.

Typical dosing for AOD 9604 is 300 mcg subcutaneously injected once per day, and the cost for a 5 mL vial is approximately $300.

ANTI-ANXIETY

Selank. This peptide was developed as a drug in Russia as a synthetic analog of another naturally produced peptide, tuftsin. Like many peptides, this one has multiple functions, but one of its analogs, Selank, has anxiolytic (anti-anxiety) and nootropic (cognitive-enhancing) properties. It appears to modulate inflammation, increase serotonin (an antidepressant neurotransmitter), increase expression of brain-derived neurotrophic factor, and inhibit the breakdown of enkephalins (peptides that act to reduce the sensation of pain, similarly to endorphins), which are one of the body's defenses against stress and pain perception. In clinical trials, Selank has been shown to be effective in treating generalized anxiety disorder without side effects of sedation, addiction, or withdrawal. Its cognitive-enhancing effect seems to result from the way it calms and reduces the brain's overactive glutamate and N-methyl-D-aspartate receptors. Some experiments also show that Selank has a positive effect on blood sugar in those with metabolic syndrome and induces an anticoagulant effect for prevention of embolic stroke.

The typical protocol for Selank is one to two sprays intranasally once per day of a 7,500 mcg/mL nasal spray costing approximately $250 for 3 mL.

Semax. Another Russian-developed drug, Semax, has anti-anxiety and cognitive-enhancing benefits. Like Selank, Semax works by increasing levels of brain-derived neurotrophic factor and serotonin while preventing the breakdown of enkephalins. It also activates the brain's dopaminergic systems to provide mood-elevating effects. Semax has been used successfully in the treatment of anxiety, depression, stroke, transient ischemic attacks, attention-deficit/hyperactivity disorder, Parkinson's disease, Alzheimer's disease, and has helped to improve immune function.

The typical protocol for Semax is one to two sprays intranasally once per day of a 7,500 mcg/mL nasal spray costing approximately $250 per 3 mL.

IMMUNE FUNCTION

Thymosin Alpha-1. This is the active ingredient in an FDA-approved drug called Zadaxin. It is the synthetic version of a naturally occurring peptide comprising twenty-eight amino acids. This substance is being studied to treat hepatitis B and C, malignant melanoma, liver cancer, DiGeorge's syndrome (a genetic disorder in which the thymus gland is not fully developed or absent), and drug-resistant tuberculosis. Some physicians are using it to treat the aftereffects (sequelae) of chronic fatigue and Lyme disease as well as autoimmune disorders including allergies. It is believed that thymosin alpha-1 modulates the immune system with its effect on T cells.

The typical protocol is to inject 450 mg subcutaneously per day. The cost for a 5 mL vial of 3,000 mcg/mL is approximately $300.

ENDOCRINE REGULATION AND TELOMERASE ACTIVATION

Epitalon. Naturally produced by the pineal gland in humans, this synthetic version functions as a bioregulator of the endocrine system. It has been shown to lengthen telomeres in human cells, but in a more complex manner than simply activating telomerase. It also reduces lipid oxidation and the formation of reactive oxygen species while modulating T cells. Epithalon has multiple anti-aging influences, including increasing sensitivity of the hypothalamus, normalizing function of the anterior pituitary, regulating gonadotropins and melatonin, and normalizing cholesterol and prolactin.

The typical dosing protocol is 10 mg via subcutaneous injection every three days for fifteen days to be performed twice per year. A 10 mg vial costs approximately $360.

"EXERCISE IN A PILL" (INJECTION)

MOTS-c. This peptide favorably affects AMPK, insulin sensitivity, and GLUT4 uptake in muscle and effectuates fat loss through its effect on fat and muscle tissue and energy regulation. In my experience, MOTS-c works considerably more effectively in those who do not exercise much and has less effect on well-trained athletes.

The protocol I suggest is to subcutaneously inject 1 mg daily. A 10 mg vial of MOTS-c costs approximately $300.

CREATING A PEPTIDE PLAN

Because so many peptides exist to treat a wide range of conditions, no single plan will fit all people. With so much research being conducted on peptides, and new products and techniques regularly emerging, what's optimal today might not be optimal tomorrow. Keeping these issues in mind, here are some recommendations for exploring peptide use for your healthspan goals.

Talk to your doctor about peptides and, if necessary, educate them about peptides in general and specific peptides in which you're interested. Some doctors will be dismissive while others will know only about their limited FDA-approved uses. Fortunately, a great number of credible studies exist that will enlighten doctors to how peptides can be used and their efficacy for specific disorders and health issues.

Ask your doctor for a peptide source if they are amenable to their use. Doctors may refer you to a regenerative medicine specialist or suggest other legal ways of obtaining the peptides you seek. Make sure the source has a track record of providing good products. An underground network has sprung up to provide peptides, and some providers are offering products of questionable source and quality. We recommend Empower Pharmacy—a federally licensed compounder (503A) and manufacturer (503B) of peptides, bioidentical hormones, and drugs for most prescriptions—and Peptide Pharmacy for those peptides that are less popular and harder to acquire.

Do your homework. Refer to the preceding list of peptides and their uses as a starting point, but also conduct some online research. I may not have covered the specific type of peptide and healthcare issue that pertains to you. It's also possible that advances have been made or new studies conducted that offer alternatives better suited to your needs since this writing.

The Rapamycin Immune System Connection

WHILE MOST OF the products and therapies discussed in this book are available for use today in some form or another, not all are easily accessible or are only reserved for very specific conditions. Rapamycin falls into the latter category. Still, it's important for you to be aware of it because of its huge potential for healing and longevity. Hundreds of studies are now being conducted to explore its potential benefits and how it can be used safely. By the time this book is published or shortly thereafter, I hope we'll have a better idea about how rapamycin's benefits can be translated from the lab to practical applications.

Until then, let's examine this amazing bacteria-inhibiting antibiotic, or macrolide.

WHAT RAPAMYCIN IS, WHAT IT DOES, AND HOW IT DOES IT

A *macrolide* is a class of naturally produced chemical compounds, of which rapamycin was discovered by scientists and isolated from bacteria found on Easter

Island in 1972. You may be familiar with macrolides if you've ever taken a type of antibiotic that includes erythromycin, azithromycin (the drug in a "Z-pack"), and clarithromycin. From a mainstream-medicine perspective, rapamycin is classified as an immunosuppressant and has been used to prevent rejection of transplanted organs, presumably by tamping down the immune response and preventing it from attacking the transplanted organ(s) it views as foreign or invasive. However, it now appears to possess what is termed an immunomodulatory function that can help restore and balance proper immune function.

Rapamycin has demonstrated significant anti-aging effects in everything from yeast to mammals, creating a great deal of interest in its potential uses, but even anti-aging doctors are often reluctant to prescribe it off-label because the doses prescribed for preventing transplant rejection can have a number of serious side effects, from raising blood sugar and cholesterol levels to causing anemia. The most significant problem, though, is rapamycin's potential reduction of immune system function; this beneficial effect for transplant patients also can put people at risk for infection, injury, or even death. As a result, scientists are working to develop products similar to rapamycin that don't cause these problems. That said, as with so many substances, the issue lies in the dosage; smaller doses administered together with the vaccines (for example, the flu vaccine) have been shown to actually enhance immune response. Both smaller doses or periodic dosing (e.g., once per week) appear to be the key in not only avoiding side effects but also getting the best result in terms of promoting better health and reducing biological age. At these "healthspan promoting" doses, the only side effect I have encountered is mouth sores that resolve when the dose of rapamycin is lowered.[31]

IMPROVING AUTOPHAGY WITH RAPAMYCIN FOR BETTER CELLULAR HEALTH

Finding the right dosage is a worthwhile effort, given rapamycin's potential to enhance healthspan. To understand this potential, let's again focus on autophagy: the cellular process by which damaged or otherwise un-useful contents of cells are broken down and recycled for a range of positive purposes. This process preserves components needed to make certain cellular structures, while cleaning up the unnecessary by-products of cellular activity, recycle dysfunctional and therefore harmful substances, providing a source of energy from within.

As this last sentence suggests, autophagy is a complex process. Think of this as a critical cleaning and recycling system that contributes to longevity and healing when it's operating at peak efficiency. By recycling the components of the cell, such as misfolded or damaged proteins, autophagy exploits the efficiencies of recycling, both in terms of the reusable components and the energy "found" in either using these components for fuel or not having to create these components from scratch.

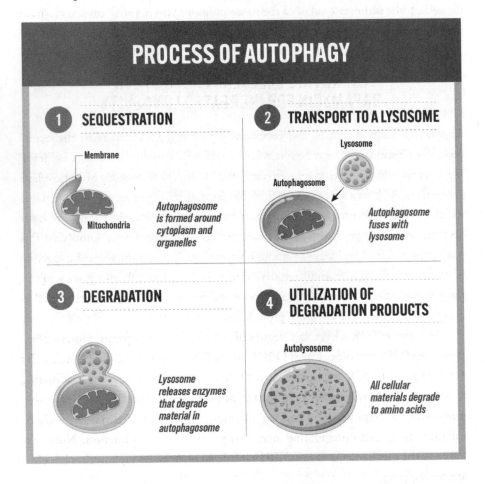

PROCESS OF AUTOPHAGY

1 SEQUESTRATION

Membrane

Mitochondria

Autophagosome is formed around cytoplasm and organelles

2 TRANSPORT TO A LYSOSOME

Lysosome

Autophagosome

Autophagosome fuses with lysosome

3 DEGRADATION

Lysosome releases enzymes that degrade material in autophagosome

4 UTILIZATION OF DEGRADATION PRODUCTS

Autolysosome

All cellular materials degrade to amino acids

Normal cellular functioning produces by-products that are either not useful for or harmful to our bodies. Autophagy gets rid of them. These by-products are analogous to the gas that results from combustion in an engine's cylinders and exits through the muffler, producing dirty exhaust particles. Autophagy helps get rid of these "particles" and offending organelles—like unneeded or irreparable mitochondria through a process actually called "mitophagy"—inside the cell, allowing our bodies to function better and more efficiently.

Not to mix metaphors, but autophagy can also be compared to keeping a kitchen in tip-top shape. If knives aren't sharpened regularly, the stove's burners and the oven aren't cleaned, counters and other surfaces aren't disinfected, food isn't stored in the refrigerator at the right temperature, and old foodstuffs aren't discarded: the ultimate quality of the meals prepared therein will suffer, as will the people consuming the meal.

IMPROVING CELLULAR ENERGY WITH RAPAMYCIN FOR INCREASED LONGEVITY

Rapamycin helps maintain this beneficial autophagy. Unfortunately, the actual process isn't simple, so let me explain how we believe it works. Let's start by defining a protein kinase, which is an enzyme that catalyzes the transfer of a phosphate group from ATP to a specific molecule. The protein kinase of relevance here is one we discussed in chapter one, mTOR (mechanistic or mammalian target of rapamycin), and it is a key term. Rapamycin inhibits mTOR, and we know that this has a positive effect on longevity, though we don't fully grasp the scientific specifics of why this is so aside from its regulation of autophagy. mTOR also plays a role in most major cell processes as a regulator of insulin and IGF-1 receptors as well as protein synthesis of cell survival, growth, and proliferation.

The way mTOR works as a regulator is through two separate protein complexes: mTOR complex 1 (mTORC1) or mTOR complex 2 (mTORC2). By inhibiting mTORC1, antagonizing mTOR promotes longevity by modulating messenger RNA translation, regulating mitochondrial function by increasing mitochondrial respiration, increasing resistance to stress and chronic age-related inflammation, and upregulating stem cell production and function. Note that many of the mechanisms of mTORC1's inhibition (and thus rapamycin's benefits) are overlapping.

Studies show that when we inhibit mTORC1, it protects us against Parkinson's disease, Alzheimer's disease, dementia, and other age-related memory and/ or learning deficits. It has shown some benefits in treating certain cancers and kidney diseases, heart disease, obesity and metabolic disorders, immune function/ dysfunction, and other disorders both related and unrelated to age.

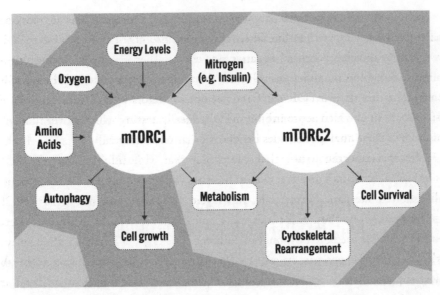

mTOR's Separate Complexes and Their Regulators and Effects

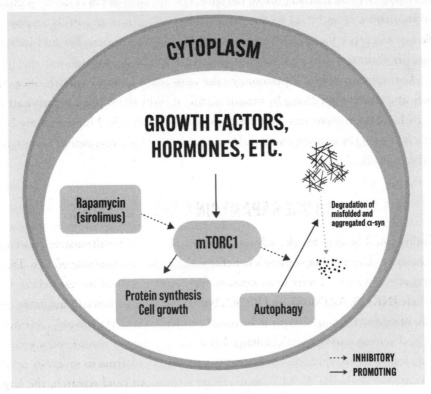

Inhibition and Promotion of mTORC1 and Its Effects

Given all these benefits, it shouldn't be surprising that researchers are working hard to develop rapamycin-like alternatives that also chemically inhibit mTOR without rapamycin's potential negative side effects. These "analogs" include everolimus, deforolimus, and temsirolimus; they target components of the mTOR pathway rather than mTOR itself and include inhibitors of S6K and agonists of 4E-BP1, both of which act to inhibit mTOR. Ideally, testing will discover that one or more of these analogs provides benefits similar to rapamycin.

It is also important to note that studies show that, while inhibition of mTORC1 is beneficial for health and can extend lifespan, inhibition of mTORC2 can actually shorten lifespan. Fortunately, rapamycin is believed to inhibit mTORC1 approximately one thousand times more potently than mTORC2, and its effect on mTORC2 is mediated by longer treatment. This helps at least partially explain why lower and/or periodic (weekly) rather than daily consistent dosing seems to yield superior results for increasing healthspan; it may also suggest a strategy for combining rapamycin or another mTORC1 inhibitor with an mTORC2 agonist (activator). Because human growth hormone (HGH) agonizes mTORC2, perhaps a combination of an HGH secretagogue with rapamycin or one of its analogs is the key to unlock the mTOR pathway to enhanced healthspan; I would look to research in the near future to substantiate and refute this hypothesis.

For what it's worth, I personally take rapamycin 6 mg by mouth once per week and ibutamoren 25 mg by mouth nightly at bedtime. While I incorporate as many healthspan increasing modalities as possible in my life, I have seen my biological age continue to improve while using this combined regimen of rapamycin and ibutamoren.

HOW TO USE RAPAMYCIN AND ITS ANALOGS

Ideally, you'll be able to take advantage of a rapamycin-like alternative relatively soon and receive all of rapamycin's benefits without the potential side effects. These alternatives, which I'll refer to as *rapalogs*, have been identified by researchers and include INK128, AZD8055, and PP242, but are not yet commercially available versions of rapamycin and have yet to be tested on mammals. Unfortunately, researching and testing rapalogs is a challenge because rapamycin is considered a generic drug, which means there isn't sufficient money for Big Pharma to invest in development. While the NIH and various private sources can fund research, the large pharmaceutical companies often are the ones driving development of new products.

If your doctor is willing to prescribe rapamycin or the analog (everolimus) off-label, you may want to take a relatively low dose to decrease the odds of side effects occurring: between 3.5 mg to 20 mg weekly for everolimus and 5 mg to 8 mg weekly for rapamycin, depending on your weight. Notably, thirty 1 mg tabs can be sourced for as low as $125. To moderate rapamycin's potential for hyperglycemic effects, you could also talk to your doctor about adding metformin. Antibiotics can also be added as needed to combat mouth ulcers, another common side effect of rapamycin.

Age also factors into your rapamycin decision. If you're twenty-six or older, then you may benefit from using rapamycin to tamp down on mTORC1 and increase cell health, but it depends on your overall physical condition and genetic factors. If you're in good shape, eat and sleep well, exercise regularly, and don't have parents or siblings who died young (from degenerative disease) or had early Alzheimer's, then you may want to wait until you get older before taking rapamycin. After age fifty, most people have accumulated a significant amount of cell damage and can benefit from rapamycin. This is all to say: it's a highly individual decision based on genetics, your current physical condition, and other factors.

The Blood Flow Molecule:
Nitric Oxide

"There may be no disease process where this miracle molecule [nitric oxide] does not have a protective role."

Louis J. Ignarro, PhD, co-recipient, Nobel Prize

NITRIC OXIDE IS a cell-signaling molecule that our bodies use for many different purposes, and the endorsement from Dr. Ignarro indicates its tremendous value. His enthusiasm for nitric oxide stems from various studies that demonstrate its positive impact on health for a variety of reasons, including its ability to relax and expand arteries, mobilize immune cells to protect against bacterial infection and cancer, facilitate the communication process within the brain, and improve erectile function.

Before going into the various uses of nitric oxide and how to take advantage of its benefits, we need to understand how this molecule works in our bodies.

NITRIC OXIDE AND ITS IMPACT ON LONGEVITY

We create nitric oxide in two different ways. First, we convert what we eat into this molecule. This process takes place in the cells within the endothelium (inner lining of blood vessels) that contain nitric oxide synthase. When we eat certain foods that are amino acid precursors, they are converted to nitric oxide. Dietary sources with these precursors include common protein-rich foods such as meats, fish, seeds, nuts, and dairy, which contain the amino acid L-arginine, as well as fruits such as watermelon, pumpkin, and cucumbers, which contain the amino acid L-citrulline.

We also produce nitric oxide by converting nitrates to nitrites to nitric oxide, through a process involving saliva and acid-resistant bacteria (bacterial nitrate reductase) that can survive in the stomach and that catalyze this process of conversion. Again, diet provides the nitrate and nitrite; leafy greens and root vegetables, especially beets, are excellent sources. Let me emphasize that, for this process to take place, we require the right bacteria to be present in the mouth and the saliva; we also require the pH of the stomach to be below 4.0. I emphasize this point because certain products can destroy bacteria or prevent the stomach from producing it, including antiseptic mouthwashes (Listerine), antacids (Tums), proton pump inhibitors (Prilosec, Prevacid, and Nexium), and histamine H_2-receptor blockers (Zantac and Pepcid AC).

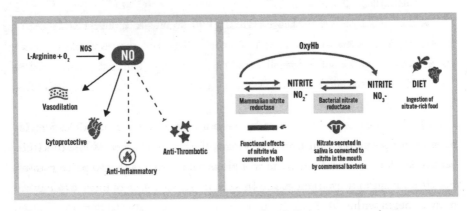

The two pathways of nitric oxide formation: (left) from nitric oxide synthase (NOS) cells within the vasculature, and (right) from bacterial conversion of ingested nitrates and nitrites to nitric oxide.

We want to keep these nitric oxide pathways open, but as we age, our nitric oxide levels naturally decrease. Failing to maintain a nitric oxide–friendly diet or being sedentary can contribute to this decrease. Later in the chapter, I'll suggest different options for increasing nitric oxide levels, but first, let's focus on the benefits of maintaining good levels.

THE NITRIC OXIDE CONNECTION TO BRAIN, HEART, AND SEXUAL FUNCTION

A person's sexual health is often a useful barometer for their metabolic or cardiovascular health and vice versa. Today, many people recognize that both diabetes and atherosclerosis are accompanied by decreased sexual health. Therefore, they have good medical motivation to seek help if they're experiencing problems in this area.

No one, regardless of age, should ignore a diminished capacity to enjoy one of life's greatest pleasures. The great news is, we have viable (though perhaps occasionally controversial) solutions to address these challenges. To name a few:

- Flibanserin (Addyi), which addresses low libido in women
- Bremelanotide, a.k.a. PT-141 (Vyleesi), which addresses libido in women and libido and erectile function in men
- Tadalafil (Cialis), sildenafil (Viagra), vardenafil (Levitra), and avanafil (Stendra), which address erectile function in men

While sexual decline with age typically corresponds to a reduction in testosterone production (in women as well as men), there are other essential considerations, such as the loss of endothelial function in the cells lining the inner walls of our vasculature that produce nitric oxide, a key component to assisting blood flow to our extremities.

Many women and men are familiar with a class of drugs called PDE-5 inhibitors, more commonly represented by Viagra, the first to market. While this intervention does work, failure rates are still pretty high, around the 30 percent mark. For these drugs to work, there has to be sufficient production of nitric oxide in the body to begin with.

Supplemental nitrite studies show that this nitric oxide pathway reduces systolic and diastolic blood pressure, improves cognitive and motor function, and reduces coronary atherosclerotic plaque in middle-aged and older adults. That said, there is emerging evidence that PDE-5 inhibition can benefit other aspects of health such as certain forms of insulin sensitivity, which could improve metabolic health and cardiovascular health, the purpose for which the drug was originally developed. Nitric oxide's role in the creation of Viagra, Cialis, and other PDE-5-inhibiting drugs best demonstrates its potential to help us heal and live longer.

During sexual arousal, nerve terminals in the penis release nitric oxide, which initiates a chain reaction that eventually produces increased blood flow into the penis—the "smooth muscles" within the penile vasculature walls relax, allowing more blood to enter. The inhibiting effect of PDE-5 increases and maintains this positive blood flow.

Because of all the research involving PDE-5-inhibiting drugs, we've discovered that nitric oxide's benefits aren't limited to sexual function. Studies demonstrate that it's effective for treating pulmonary hypertension, diabetes, Alzheimer's disease and other central nervous system disorders, congestive heart failure, peripheral artery disease, Raynaud's syndrome, benign prostatic hypertrophy, ocular diseases, and altitude sickness.

WHERE ARE YOU SEXUALLY?

Gaining insight into sexual health is now very much a clinically standardized process, which one can start right in the privacy of one's own home. Find a moment to take the Golombok-Rust Inventory of Sexual Satisfaction and the Changes in Sexual Functioning Questionnaire. Both of these self-reported evaluations can offer a valuable perspective on one's sexual health, and act as a point of departure for a deeper discussion with your physician. And yes, even cosmetic procedures can have a beneficial effect on sexual health and pleasure.

Dr. Eugene Shippen, my colleague and friend, made me aware of a fascinating study published in the journal *Heart* (August 2017) of 43,145 men under eighty years of age (mean age of sixty-four) who had been hospitalized after having heart attacks, but did not have prior histories of cardiac problems.[32] A percentage of these men received testosterone replacement therapy and statin therapy. Of these men, 7.1 percent received medication for erectile dysfunction—most of them were given a PDE-5 inhibitor. After a little more than three years, a follow-up study revealed that the men who received one dose weekly of the PDE-5 inhibitor had a reduced mortality rate of 34 percent, those who received two to five doses weekly saw a mortality rate reduction of 53 percent, and those who received more than five doses weekly had a mortality rate reduction of 81 percent.[33]

While this study in isolation certainly has its limitations—we can't conclude that everyone who receives more than five doses of a PDE-5 inhibitor weekly will reduce their mortality rate so sharply—we can recognize that this is an extraordinary result that adds to the conclusions of other studies that demonstrate the benefits of nitric oxide.

In fact, Dr. Shippen informed me of another study, this one published in the *World Journal of Diabetes* (March 15, 2017), which identified a significant reduction in mortality among those treated with PDE-5 inhibitors versus those who didn't receive this treatment. The study also reported that the mortality rate was further reduced when PDE-5 inhibitors were combined with statin use and testosterone replacement therapy.

DIY WAYS TO BOOST NITRIC OXIDE

Taking advantage of what we've learned about nitric oxide isn't difficult. Here are some simple steps anyone, male or female, can take to gain the mortality reduction benefit and other positive outcomes of what Dr. Ignarro referred to as a "miracle molecule":

- *Eat a lot of nitrate- and nitrite-containing foods:* These include beets, celery, leafy green vegetables, turnips, radishes, onions, and garlic. While preserved meats do contain nitrates (in the form of sodium nitrates), it's much better to obtain your nitrates/nitrites from vegetables because consumption of excess sodium nitrate may be linked to cancer. Vegetables, however, contain antioxidants that can help prevent nitrates from morphing into cancer-causing substances like nitrosamine.

- **Supplement with precursors to nitric oxide:** If one does not have extant coronary artery disease or other form of endothelial dysfunction that would hinder the production of nitric oxide from the amino acids L-arginine and L-citrulline, then one can supplement with 2 g to 4 g of either per day costing at most \$5/day. Otherwise, and for a more powerful method, supplement with a clinically proven nitric oxide product that actually generates nitric oxide gas. These can be found in the form of orally disintegrating lozenges or through fermented boot root powders (my favorite can be found at http://www.no2u.com).

- *Take a small dose of a PDE-5 inhibitor daily:* For instance, take 5 mg to 10 mg of Cialis. PDE-5 inhibitors may be covered by insurance, reducing the cost further.
- *Increase your testosterone levels:* Get an adequate amount of sleep, exercise regularly, eat a balanced diet, and reduce stress. Or, instead, undergo testosterone replacement therapy.
- *Take a statin or a statin-like product:* Obtain a prescription, or eat foods such as red yeast rice, if you've been diagnosed with coronary heart disease or are at high risk for it, to benefit from the combination of PDE-5 inhibitors and statins.

The takeaway here is that nitric oxide is essential to optimal health and improving healthspan, and you can improve your odds against dying from various causes by using one or more of these tactics to increase and preserve nitric oxide levels. They're relatively inexpensive ways to capitalize on its significant benefits.

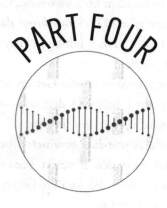

PART FOUR

Living Longer and Better with Hormones

Bioidentical Hormone Replacement Therapy

AT AGE THIRTY-FIVE on average, perimenopause (for women) and periandropause (for men) begin and people experience a decrease in hormone production. Stress can also catalyze hormone deficiencies.

No matter the cause, the symptoms of decreasing hormone levels are the same and may include a loss of libido and energy, a diminished sense of well-being, less ability to control body composition (i.e., difficulty getting rid of a stubborn layer of fat around the middle), decreased cognitive function, anxiety, and insomnia—just to name a few.

These issues may not seem as significant as the symptoms of major diseases, but from a healthspan perspective, they are crucial. A loss of libido can create a rift in your relationship with the person you love. Frequently feeling sluggish can stop you from getting necessary exercise. Less specifically, hormonal deficiencies can make you feel like you're not yourself, like you've become an old man or woman seemingly overnight.

This is when bioidentical hormone replacement therapy (BHRT) is very useful. We've learned how to restore hormones to youthful levels and restore patients' vigor and vitality with few side effects (which we've also learned how to manage). Let's begin with an explanation of what BHRT is and how it works in our bodies.

CHEATING HORMONAL DECLINE IN BOTH MEN AND WOMEN

On the surface, the logic of BHRT is simple: we lose hormones as we age, but now we can restore these hormone levels to where they were when we were younger. It's not just about numerical hormone levels, though. As I'm fond of saying, we treat the patient, not the numbers. The goal is to restore that sense of well-being, energy, libido, and ability to control body composition, among other aforementioned abilities and feelings.

The word *bioidentical* in BHRT is important, since we're focusing on hormones the body produces naturally throughout life. These include sex hormones made from cholesterol (testosterone and estrogen) as well as those made from protein (thyroid and growth hormones). The hormones used in BHRT are made synthetically in labs, but they're the same structure as those synthesized by our bodies, as opposed to hormones that aren't bioidentical and are obtained from other sources like horse urine. In managing signs and symptoms of estrogen deficiency, human bioidentical estrogens such as estriol and estradiol are used to avoid the risks associated with estrones and non-bioidentical hormones.

BHRT is designed to control or eliminate symptoms that come with having low levels of certain hormones. Specifically, deficiency in the following hormones produces these symptoms:

- *Thyroid hormones.* Chills, fatigue, sluggishness, dry skin and hair.
- *Testosterone.* Low libido and energy, diminished sense of well-being, body composition changes such as loss of muscle mass and gain of fat mass, erectile dysfunction, cognition difficulties, slow recovery after exercise, and insomnia are other symptoms.
- *Estrogen.* Hot flashes, vaginal dryness, night sweats, anxiety.
- *DHEA.* Decrease in energy, reduced immune function, increased systemic inflammation.

- ***Pregnenolone.*** Decrease in cognitive function and ability to appreciate color.
- ***Progesterone.*** Decreasing health of vasculature, anxiety, insomnia.

Many people don't recognize these symptoms as stemming from hormone deficiency. Because they often develop gradually, people ascribe them to a particular event ("I haven't been getting much sleep, that must be why I'm lacking energy") or resign themselves to the aging process and figure there's not much they can do about these symptoms beyond taking a pain reliever or drinking a double espresso for energy.

While aging is the primary reason we experience hormone deficiencies, stress can accelerate the decline. Most people start losing hormones at age thirty-five, but people under significant stress can start losing them even earlier. Given the society in which we live and the pressure many of us are under, it's not surprising that people today lose hormones faster than hundreds of years ago in an agrarian society where, aside from concerns about wolves eating your sheep and other singular, calamitous events, stress was not the constant that it is for many people in the twenty-first century.

Lack of deep sleep can also hamper hormone production. For instance, the anterior pituitary gland releases growth hormone and prolactin, and the pineal gland produces melatonin, when we're sound asleep. If we're not sleeping well because of aging or stress, we're creating less than the optimal amount of needed hormones.

We also can stress ourselves physically. Over-exercising can stress the body and accelerate hormone loss. In my experience, athletes typically don't produce more testosterone (or other hormones) than the average person, contrary to what many people believe. In fact, they may produce less if they place too much stress on their bodies by working out harder and longer than they should. It's not always over-exercise that's the problem but, rather, under-recovery. We may work out regularly and effectively, but we don't recover properly. We fail to get adequate sleep, don't eat or hydrate properly, and fail to do stretches or use other techniques to help our soft tissues loosen after intense exercise. All of these factors can contribute to hormone loss.

The term *sick thyroid* refers to how the thyroid gland reduces its hormone production because of overwork. Many years ago in human societies, the thyroids of people who couldn't hunt and gather because of injury or illness reduced hormone production in order to save energy. Today, if we overtax our bodies, the thyroid responds similarly.

Doctors rely on two methods to determine if hormone deficiency is occurring. First (and foremost), we look for the signs and symptoms just described, factoring in the age of the patients and how much stress they're under. Second, we take blood samples to measure hormone levels that support why an individual might be experiencing their symptoms.

Though hormone replacement isn't the only option when we determine a deficiency exists, it's often the best one. Let's take a look at how replacement works relative to three specific hormones.

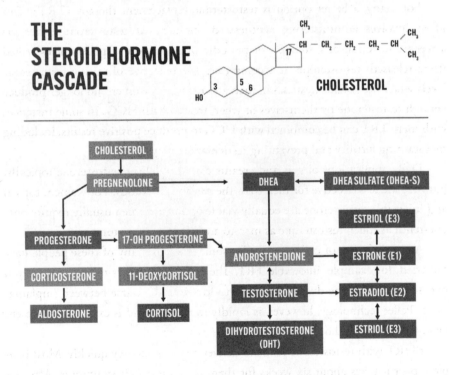

TESTOSTERONE DEFICIENCY

Imagine, if you will, Jim, a forty-three-year-old male, who has blood tests and symptoms that may indicate he is testosterone deficient. Jim is also under a lot of stress—he just lost his job and is in the middle of a divorce. Given all these factors, it may be that his pituitary gland is failing to send signals to his testicles to produce sufficient amounts of testosterone. One way we can stimulate the testicles to produce more testosterone is by using a substance called human chorionic gonadotropin (HCG), which mimics the body's use of luteinizing hormone to signal the need for more testosterone. This treatment involves injecting yourself with a solution of HCG at least twice weekly, with other practical considerations including reconstituting the HCG and keeping it refrigerated. However, it is often the problem that, at forty-three, Jim's testicles will either not respond sufficiently or, for reasons we don't quite know, even a significant response by the testicles to produce endogenous testosterone is not enough to correct the deficiency and relieve his symptoms entirely.

For many, a better option is testosterone replacement therapy (TRT). This often involves administering synthesized, bioidentical testosterone either via a weekly injection of a solution or periodic implantation of pellets of esterified (time-released) testosterone. It accomplishes the objective of raising testosterone levels when the gonads (testicles in men and ovaries in women) no longer produce enough testosterone by themselves or when treated with HCG. In some instances with men, TRT can be combined with HCG to produce positive results, including maintaining fertility and preventing testicular atrophy.

Daily applications of gels and creams can also deliver testosterone topically, but they are less effective for men than the previous methods. For women, topical and injectable testosterone are equally viable options; women usually require only one-tenth as much testosterone as men to address their symptoms.

Administration of pellets works for some, though many of these people have not tried, for example, injectable TRT. The issue with pellets remains an uneven release of testosterone during the three-to-four-month course between implantations. Pellet technology, however, is rapidly improving and is expected to present an equally successful option for TRT in the near future.

BHRT with testosterone tends to deliver results relatively quickly. Most people report it takes about six weeks for them to resolve their symptoms. After six weeks, men with libido or erectile dysfunction issues notice that they're waking up with erections, their previous lethargy ebbs, and they're energized enough to go to the gym and work out. Women talk about how they feel reenergized and aren't experiencing their routine post-lunch energy crash. Both find that their renewed sense of well-being translates into less insomnia and better, deeper sleep.

It takes longer for BHRT to affect body composition—at least three and a half months. This delay is because it requires the initial six weeks to "kick in" followed by at least a month for testosterone to rebuild muscle in response to exercise, good nutrition, and proper rest. Another month is needed for results to become visible, for muscle to begin to raise caloric requirements and assist in delving into accumulated fat stores for energy.

TRT isn't a magic pill that works on its own; testosterone doesn't build muscle unless you do the work. You need to leverage the replaced hormone through exercise, good nutrition, and proper sleep. Conversely, we have patients who come to us insisting that they're doing all the right things and they haven't been able to alter their body composition; it's only when they combine all these good habits with TRT that they see the results.

Replacing testosterone may also confer a host of disease-fighting benefits. Studies dating back to the 1950s have associated low testosterone levels with CAD, diabetes, colon cancer, osteoporosis, and prostate cancer. Though it's impossible to claim that TRT can prevent or treat these diseases without further studies, it's an area that bears watching. In a relatively small study (fifteen participants), "bipolar" TRT (periodic treatment and stoppage) has been used to treat prostate cancer successfully and showed that TRT can slow, stop, or reverse osteoporosis when combined with weight-bearing exercise, nutrition, and rest.

Patients always ask if there's a downside to replacing testosterone, partly because of a flawed study from the 1940s that concluded testosterone treatment caused prostate cancer. Despite the fact that this study was faulty—there were only three people in the study, two of whom should have been excluded in hindsight!—and that other studies have not supported its conclusions, the taint of a supposedly negative study lingers. Similarly, rumors circulated that said women who take testosterone turned into muscle-bound hulks. Again, these rumors are false; with the right dose and good exercise and nutrition habits, women are no more likely to turn into the *Incredible Hulk* than men are. People control their own body narratives, not a body-transforming pill.

If there's a downside to testosterone replacement, it's that this hormone can convert to estrogen. While necessary for both men and women, excess amounts of estrogen can cause water and fat retention along with moodiness and irascibility, may promote estrogen-sensitive cancers in women, and can activate genes for prostate cancer that all men carry. This last effect sounds ominous; consider that today in the US, all men have prostate cancer by age eighty-two, but it's often slow growing and may not have the opportunity to become a life-threatening problem, as they're more likely to die of something else before this cancer can reach its end stages. Perhaps more importantly, we know that by controlling excess estrogen, particularly the two from the estrone family of estrogens, we can prevent the activation of these cancer genes. A urine or blood test (2/16 alpha-hydroxyestrone) can help determine one's proclivity to developing estrogen-sensitive cancers. We also know that consumption of cruciferous vegetables like broccoli, cauliflower, Brussels sprouts, and so forth can improve this ratio by promoting conversion from estrone family (specifically the 4-hydroxyestrone and 16-alpha-hydroxyestrone) to the harmless and necessary estrogens such as estriol, estradiol, and 2-hydroxyestrone. If you do not enjoy those vegetables, you can take supplemental indole-3-carbinol or DIM, both of which are derived from these cruciferous vegetables and can prevent this conversion.

There are a number of other possible, purportedly annoying effects of adding testosterone: from enlarging a woman's clitoris (when excessive amounts of testosterone are used; this is related more to its conversion to dihydrotestosterone than testosterone) to activating the gene for body hair growth, male pattern baldness, and acne. Some women notice topical hair growth when they apply testosterone to their skin. When this happens, many women aren't particularly concerned, either because it's not noticeable or because the benefits of treatment far outweigh this side effect. But these potential side effects are genetically based and not directly related to testosterone, but rather to a metabolite from testosterone called dihydrotestosterone (DHT). If you notice any of the aforementioned side effects, they can all be reversed by simply blocking the conversion from testosterone into dihydrotestosterone. This used to be done for women—on TRT or not—with the use of a diuretic drug called spironolactone, which carries a side effect of inhibiting the conversion from testosterone to DHT. Nowadays, we use a single drug, finasteride (a.k.a. Propecia or Proscar, depending upon the strength) for men and women to block the enzyme, 5-alpha reductase, that converts testosterone into DHT. Any side effects from this overproduction of DHT resolve typically within six weeks after starting on finasteride. Otherwise, if these effects surface, they can also be reversed by simply stopping TRT within as many as six months of the side effects' appearance.

In addition, when men start on testosterone replacement therapy, they are given another drug to control the conversion from testosterone into excess estrogen. While excess estrogen can result in water retention, fat retention, moodiness and irascibility, gynecomastia (growth of breast tissue), and activation of certain genes that all men carry for prostate cancer, some estrogen is essential for heart, brain, and joint health in both men and women. We can modulate this conversion by also giving men (and women) an inhibitory drug that prevents the enzyme aromatase from converting testosterone to estrogen.

ANABOLIC STEROIDS

Most often associated with abuse in bodybuilders or cheating in sports, anabolic steroids leverage the body's ability to recover after exercise, particularly to help build muscle through high-intensity efforts followed by appropriate nutrition and adequate rest. I mention it here because, despite its reputation, it can be a very useful drug when used appropriately. A steroid is a hormone naturally produced by the body from cholesterol; types of steroid include estrogen, progesterone, DHEA, and pregnenolone as well as testosterone. An anabolic steroid is an unnatural molecule designed to leverage the body's ability to accrete muscle mass and is usually derived from a molecule resembling testosterone or dihydrotestosterone. I choose the word *leverage* purposefully because many mistakenly believe that if one simply takes an anabolic steroid they can, like it or not, end up looking like Arnold Schwarzenegger. On the contrary: one must "do the work"—training right, eating right, and sleeping/resting right—in order to have a bodybuilder's physique. Still, use of anabolic steroids amplifies the ability to make muscle, as instigated by doing the appropriate and necessary work.

One of the leading (fourth most common) causes of death in the United States is accidental death; of those, falls rank third. Somewhat misleading in this statistic is that, while the actual fall may not be the cause of death, in the elderly, the deterioration of health after being hospitalized and not being able to move or otherwise function normally often leads to death. If they didn't die from the fall, the resulting rapid decline in health from immobility or pneumonia while hospitalized killed them. Anabolic steroids can be used to help strengthen the infirm and frail in order to help prevent death from accidental falls (or to prevent falls in general). Their use in both critical and normal situations wherein muscle mass and strength have deteriorated, thus damaging healthspan, can help promote health more powerfully. One cannot perform his or her daily exercise and otherwise enjoy life if one does not have the muscle, strength, or energy to do so. That leads to the spiraling downward into "old age" that all of us want to avoid, if we don't actively dread it.

A Sampling of Steroid Molecules with Anabolic Properties

ESTROGEN DEFICIENCY

When women experience estrogen deficiency in addition to testosterone deficiency, one possible replacement tactic is simply testosterone. Because testosterone is an estrogen precursor, enough estrogen is often converted from replaced testosterone to alleviate estrogen deficiency, especially in younger women. This may be all that's needed to restore estrogen to normal levels. If replacing testosterone alone isn't effective, we add estrogen to the mix. Generally, we start with a minimal dose, the smallest amount possible that helps resolve symptoms. If that isn't enough, we bump up the dose slightly until it starts working. Once the symptoms disappear, we start reducing the dose to reach the smallest amount that is still effective.

We usually combine two types of estrogen: 80 percent estriol and 20 percent estradiol (estriol is the weaker of the two). Though estriol is not associated with estrogen-sensitive cancers and may in fact be anticarcinogenic, estradiol has been associated with cancer, but likely indirectly, through its conversion to certain estrones ("bad" forms of estrogen). Nonetheless, no studies show that this particular combination *causes* cancer. For women still concerned about this possibility, doctors can add substances that block the conversion to the "bad" estrones; eating cruciferous vegetables can also help prevent this conversion. Regardless, cruciferous vegetables and taking a supplement like DIM is a good idea even if you're not undergoing BHRT, since women's bodies naturally begin converting their good estrogen into bad as well as not converting their bad into good as they age.

HUMAN GROWTH HORMONE

This protein-based hormone is different from the others we've discussed; it's actually a peptide, composed of 191 different amino acids, and it's produced by the pituitary gland. Its name is a bit of a misnomer. While it is used to stimulate growth of the long bones of children, it is not used to catalyze growth in adults. Instead, many adults request HGH for reduction of fat or for its regeneration capabilities in helping repair tendons, ligaments, and skin. The last one is particularly popular, since HGH improves the thickness of the dermal layer of skin and helps retain water within cells (rather than outside of cells), resulting in better skin turgor and appearance. As humans, we start out in life composed of about 70 percent water, but if we live long enough, we may only be 50 percent water in our senior years—the dryness causes our skin to look wrinkled and old. HGH can address this issue.

In the majority of cases, however, BHRT using testosterone or estrogen can address many of these issues effectively—and legally. HGH has only been approved by the FDA for a handful of uses, mostly related to lack of normal growth in children. In adults, it's approved for muscle-wasting diseases caused by HIV, short bowel syndrome, and HGH deficiency resulting from a tumor (or its treatment). While some doctors may prescribe HGH for non-FDA approved uses (illegally, as HGH is the only FDA-approved drug that is not approved for off-label use), and some patients may travel to other countries to receive HGH injections, we can increase our HGH safely and less expensively by taking peptides, which stimulate the pituitary gland to produce more HGH.

For instance, growth hormone secretagogues are substances (usually peptides) that can be injected subcutaneously. Peptidomimetics (a fancy way of saying they work like a peptide, but aren't one) like ibutamoren (previously mentioned in chapter twelve) come in pill form and are far less expensive than injectable HGH, which often costs $2,000 monthly at a minimum. Secretagogues are about one-tenth the cost of HGH, and those in pill form are more convenient than injectable HGH, which also has to be refrigerated. Even better, these substances are legal to prescribe and use.

FREQUENTLY ASKED QUESTIONS ABOUT HORMONE REPLACEMENT

Hormone replacement therapy, more than many of the other treatments, products, and devices discussed in this book, has been the subject of controversy. Actually, the controversy is more in mainstream medicine than in anti-aging medical research circles, where the value of BHRT is well known—though, as we'll see, debate exists on the best treatment approach. Some of the controversy is financial, as insurance plans often don't cover BHRT. It's also the subject of some debate about its most effective uses and how to maximize results. Patients often ask me questions about BHRT—especially testosterone replacement—so I'm going to share their questions and concerns with you.

I'VE HEARD THAT BHRT IS DANGEROUS; WHAT EVIDENCE IS THERE THAT IT'S A SAFE THERAPY?

Drs. Larry Lipshultz, Eugene Shippen, Abraham Morgentaler, John Lee, and Jonathan Wright are five answers to this question. These are all esteemed US physicians and researchers who are leaders in the BHRT field and have conducted extensive studies and written papers on the subject. Look them up and you'll find their conclusions about BHRT's safety.

I recognize that it's natural to be concerned about BHRT's safety. If you watch ESPN especially, you've probably seen a commercial for a class action lawsuit that asks viewers to call the advertiser (a law firm) if they've taken testosterone. I have a lifelong friend who is a personal injury attorney and TRT patient; when I asked him about this lawsuit, he said that it wasn't about medicine but about money that could be gained by citing a recently published study that had concluded testosterone replacement could be unsafe. Even though *many* physicians criticized this study and others that followed, some attorneys saw a big payday and pounced. In fact, both the studies and the peer-reviewed journals that published them were criticized for what was clearly irresponsible and, frankly, *bad science*.[34]

WILL TESTOSTERONE REPLACEMENT HELP INCREASE FERTILITY AND CHANCES OF CONCEPTION?

This question has a few different answers. First, women should not undergo testosterone replacement therapy when pregnant. Testosterone is an androgen and, as such, might affect the fetus adversely. Therefore, in all stages of pregnancy, but especially the early ones, avoid testosterone replacement. On the other hand, in some cases, testosterone replacement could be useful in preparation for becoming pregnant. It can be used to leverage the restoration of health of women and the uterus.

For men, testosterone is essential for producing sperm, but it's a complex process that leads to confusion about the value of testosterone replacement. It is true that testosterone replacement can result in a reduction in the number of sperm produced or temporary infertility (defined via semen analysis as fewer than 15 *million* sperm per milliliter of semen) because it affects the pituitary's perception of the amount of testosterone needed. The exogenously added testosterone is registered by the pituitary as sufficient so that it can send fewer signals to the testicles to produce less (part of a process called a "negative feedback loop"), ultimately resulting in fewer sperm. Though this infertility can be reversed by stopping testosterone replacement, many men don't want to stop it because of all the other benefits they receive from TRT.

One solution, therefore, can be the use of HCG, which I discussed earlier in the chapter. Used in conjunction with testosterone replacement, it can help the body keep producing endogenous testosterone, specifically intratesticular testosterone, sufficient to prime the process for creating additional sperm.

Another option for men is to bank sperm for later use before beginning TRT. Not only does this provide an additional backup reservoir of sperm for conception, it also gives you a store of "younger" sperm that you can use as you become older—yes, younger sperm has been shown to be more viable. Banking sperm does not mean that this sperm *must* be used—fertility specialists typically reserve using banked sperm only for when sexual intercourse fails to result in conception—but it can alleviate any worries about fertility being an issue down the road, whether secondary to TRT or stemming from any other negative influence. I should add that in my years of medical practice, I have never seen a case of a man who has become infertile secondary to TRT not regaining his fertility either by adding HCG to his regimen or discontinuing TRT.

ARE THERE NEGATIVE EFFECTS IF YOU STOP TESTOSTERONE REPLACEMENT THERAPY? IS THERE VALUE IN REDUCING THE TESTOSTERONE DOSE TO LIMIT ANY NEGATIVE EFFECTS?

In some instances, young men and women cycle on and off replacement therapy when they're using it for cosmetic or athletic purposes, wanting to keep their natural production of testosterone at an optimal level, and for procreation purposes while not becoming "dependent" on TRT before it is "necessary." As far as we know, there are no negative effects of this start-and-stop methodology, except in cases where men and women are still developing their hypothalamic-pituitary-adrenal axis (i.e., usually before the age of twenty-six years). We know from experience with TRT as well as hormonal birth control methods that disrupting the hormones during the development of this hormone-regulating axis can affect its proper development and result in lifetime deficiencies or imbalances thereafter. For older men who aren't concerned about their fertility, there's no need to stop. Still, some do out of an abundance of caution; they believe that if a risk exists, they're limiting it by cycling on and off or by reducing their testosterone dose. There really isn't much point in doing so and the risk in stopping or reducing the dose is that you also reduce the beneficial effects of the therapy.

The body has what amounts to a hormone thermostat. If we add external testosterone, the body reduces its own production in order to maintain its preexisting level, harkening back to the aforementioned "negative feedback loop." That's why, when patients request a relatively modest or conservative starting dose, we explain that nothing but a full dose will work, because our body's hormone thermostat will compensate for the relatively smaller dose of exogenous testosterone by reducing its own production commensurately. A simple way to consider this issue is as a numerical value. If we know that the optimal level represents a "10," then, whether you are starting from a "1" or a "4," you will need what amounts to a dose of "10" to reach "10." In truth, the physiology is not quite as linear, but for purposes of our discussion, it is pretty close.

HOW MUCH ADDED TESTOSTERONE IS NEEDED FOR IT TO BE EFFECTIVE? IS THE AMOUNT DIFFERENT FOR MEN AND WOMEN?

We have studies from the 1950s showing that for men, the recommended thera-peutic dose is one in which the "total testosterone" assay does not fall below 800 nanograms per deciliter. For women, the amount should not fall below three times the upper limit considered normal, or approximately 150 nanograms per deciliter. We now know that *free testosterone*, rather than *total testosterone*, is a better measure because *free testosterone* is actually available in the body for use. For men, we gener-ally aim for no less than measures in the high twenties in picograms per milliliter; for women, no less than about four picograms per milliliter.

Let me emphasize again that, as a physician, I don't treat numbers; I treat the patient. People are individuals with highly individualized responses to treatment. These numbers are meant to guide the physician toward the optimal dose for the patient, but this dose may vary considerably. I have patients who come into my office for follow-up with levels well below those I have mentioned, but who are ecstatic with the results of therapy. Others definitely notice the decrease in symp-tom resolution when their testosterone levels drop a day or two before their next dose. We adjust the dose and frequency based upon the resolution of their signs and symptoms rather than just the testosterone assay number.

On October 1, 2015, Dr. Abraham Morgentaler chaired an international group of eighteen experts from eleven countries who met in Prague, Czech Republic, to develop a consensus of nine resolutions regarding male hypogonadism (low testos-terone). Published in 2016, the nine unanimously approved resolutions address the misconceptions and answer many questions about TRT.[35]

As mentioned, doctors monitor testosterone levels through blood work to help ensure we're achieving and maintaining the optimal levels for resolving their prob-lem as a result of deficiency. This means measuring not only testosterone levels but also the conversion of testosterone into estrogen or dihydrotestosterone, for exam-ple, and other metabolites of testosterone. We continue to monitor levels of testos-terone and other metabolites over time because, as the body ages and changes, so does its metabolism of testosterone. After six weeks of TRT, most people start to feel its benefits, and their symptoms start to abate if not completely resolve. Many patients go through what I call a "honeymoon period" as the testosterone kicks in and the body's receptors for testosterone remain upregulated from the period of low testosterone leading up to TRT. The human body is pretty amazing in that, when it cannot produce enough of a hormone, it adapts by upregulating receptors for that hormone. During the period before the body recognizes the now relative overabundance of testosterone, the patient often feels better than ever, until the receptors are eventually downregulated to a more relatively normal number.

About ninety days after beginning therapy, patients are evaluated at what I refer to as their new baseline for TRT. We do the labs at this point, look at the levels of testosterone and various metabolites and precursors, and—most importantly— evaluate how people are feeling contrasted with how they were feeling before treatment. Though higher testosterone levels usually don't cause issues directly, as the titer of testosterone rises higher than what the body considers within the homeostatic range of "normal," more of it is metabolized to other metabolites like estrogens and dihydrotestosterone in an effort to reduce the testosterone level. If any of these conversions are an issue, we can add the previously mentioned inhibitors. In men with a genetic disposition to male pattern baldness, too much dihydrotestosterone can contribute to this condition by accelerating head hair loss, so for these patients we make sure levels don't climb too high.

Still, testosterone treatment isn't as level dependent as it is for thyroid hormone, where we're looking for a sweet spot between too high and too low. With testosterone—using typical TRT doses—this sweet spot is not of concern; rather, we seek to maintain levels above a therapeutic minimum threshold. The biggest problem is if the level of testosterone dips too low, patients won't realize the benefits of the therapy.

IS TESTOSTERONE REPLACEMENT THERAPY VIABLE OVER THE LONG TERM? ARE THERE ISSUES I SHOULD CONSIDER MOVING FORWARD?

It is viable long term, and we have many patients who have been doing BHRT for years. Still, as with all treatments, some cautions exist.

For both men and women, it's important to do blood tests to determine testosterone and related hormone levels regularly (at least annually) after therapy starts. Again, while we're not concerned about excessive testosterone with replacement dosages, we want to make sure the treatment hasn't resulted in the testosterone converting into excessive dihydrotestosterone or estrogens (particularly certain estrones), especially if a patient is experiencing any of the aforementioned potential side effects, as well as to be proactive in limiting side effects and potentiating estrogen-sensitive cancers. Again, let me emphasize this point: these hormones—testosterone, dihydrotestosterone, estriol, estradiol—do not cause cancer, but they may "fuel" existing cancer. Dihydrotestosterone, for example, does not cause prostate cancer in men but can fuel it once it is present.

Patients should check with their doctors ninety days after starting TRT and each year thereafter, especially if their circumstances (such as differences in lifestyle, added stressors, etc.) are changing. Most times at follow-up there will be little or no change to dosing, but it's a good idea to monitor the most obvious signs and symptoms for changes between follow-ups: libido, energy, and so on. We also want to make sure there are no unwanted side effects and, if there are, address how we can control them.

Last, consider that a 2017 Swedish study of almost 44,000 people concluded that three types of treatments, when taken together, can reduce all-cause mortality by an astonishing 81 percent: statins, PDE-5 inhibitors, and TRT. That's compelling evidence that this type of therapy, TRT, has great value; not just for helping people look and feel good, but for enabling them to live longer.

Costs of this treatment aren't high; if not covered by insurance, the monthly expense for injectable testosterone for a male is around $100 and for a female around $30. The monthly cost of topical testosterone therapy for both men and women is approximately $60. As mentioned in chapter twelve, we recommend Empower Pharmacy, a federally licensed compounding pharmacy based in Houston, Texas, as a reliable and fairly priced source of bioidentical hormones. By the time of publication, they will be considered the largest compounder in the world, with facilities built by the same companies and to the same standards as those of the major pharmaceutical manufacturers.

WHY IS THERE SO MUCH EMPHASIS ON TESTOSTERONE REPLACEMENT THERAPY VERSUS OTHER HORMONES?

Because it has the broadest use for the most patients, at least among my patients. BHRT/TRT works for people of all genders and ages, especially once natural production of testosterone has declined. It addresses many healthspan-related issues, from appearance to energy to sex. In addition, it's especially useful for people going through tough times. It helps foster a sense of well-being, giving patients the stamina and energy necessary to deal with life challenges. Plus, a Harvard study demonstrated the connection between higher levels of testosterone and success.[36]

Given all the positives of testosterone and BHRT, you would think that it would be more widely embraced by the public and the medical community. The problem, though, is that there isn't a lot of money to be made with these products, and money often drives awareness. Pharmaceutical companies create tremendous awareness for their products through advertising to the public and in their communications with the healthcare community, but they're looking for products on which they can get patents and recoup their R&D costs, not drugs like bioidentical hormones.

I HAVE HEARD THAT TAKING ESTROGEN CAN CAUSE BLOOD CLOTS AND CANCER. SHOULDN'T I BE CONCERNED WITH BIOIDENTICAL HORMONE REPLACEMENT OF ESTROGEN?

The Women's Health Initiative (WHI) study of more than 161,000 participants, launched in 1992, had a significant impact on women's health and medical interventions. However, one unfortunate result was its failure to recognize that there are monumental and inarguable differences between bioidentical estrogens and those derived from horses. Without noting these differences, the WHI study drew conclusions that estrogen replacement causes an increase in cancer and stroke incidence. As mentioned, we know that the problematic estrogens are in the estrone group, specifically 16-alpha-hydroxyestrone and 4-hydroxyestrone, because these estrogens are much more powerful in effect than 2-hydroxyestrone and other estrogens like estriol. Equilin, derived from horse urine and used to make the product that most women in the WHI study used, has an estrogen effect at least one thousand times more potent than any human estrogen. So, it comes as no surprise that estrogen replacement with this molecule resulted in an increased incidence of certain estrogen-sensitive cancers (e.g., endometrial) and stroke.

While no studies have been undertaken to evaluate similar risks using bioidentical estrogens, I have seen no evidence to show that they do. That said, given our aforementioned understanding of estrones and hormone physiology—specifically that, as we age, we convert less of the "bad" (more potent and carcinogenic) estrogens to the "good" (less potent and potentially anticarcinogenic) estrogens, and

vice versa—I suggest that women (and men) consume plenty of cruciferous vegetables (e.g., broccoli, cauliflower, Brussels sprouts) and/or supplement with DIM
and I3C, the protective ingredients sought from these vegetables to promote conversion from "bad' to "good" estrogens. In addition, supplementing with omega-3
fish oil, rich in fatty acids (dosage of 2 grams or more by mouth per day), makes
blood platelets less "sticky" and decreases risk of stroke for anyone (whether on
estrogen replacement therapy or not).

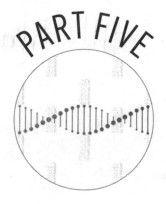

Cheating Death with Technology, Analytics, and Action

Cheating Death with Early Detection and Diagnosis

MANY DISEASES ARE curable, or at least manageable, if caught early, and many of us can improve our healthspan if we monitor our signs and symptoms regularly. As much as the healthcare profession emphasizes early screening for some illnesses—colon, breast, and prostate cancer and heart disease especially—it fails to emphasize early detection and treatment across the board. More to the point, doctors and other healthcare professionals fail to capitalize on many of the early-detection tools available. Therefore, before I introduce you to some of these tools, you need to understand why your doctor may not be recommending them.

This emphasis on screening over early detection and treatment is evident in the topics of papers presented at typical cancer conferences. Screenings such as mammograms or colonoscopies are typically only sensitive enough to discover disease after the fact, whereas early detection tests such as Time of Flight PET/CT, multiparametric MRI, GRAIL, and RGCC are sensitive enough to detect cancer at stage 0, prior to its classification as a formal disease state. Also, many insurance companies do not even cover treatment until the cancer diagnosis reaches stage II or beyond. *Why?* Cells are mutating all the time in the human body, but the body has mechanisms—some of which we have discussed—that correct for these mutations either by fixing or, more often, destroying the mutated cell. As a result, identifying mutations may produce what are essentially false positives.

Let's say I have a number of mutations slightly above whatever level is determined as "cancer." After I'm tested, my doctor may say, "Dr. McClain, you have been diagnosed with pancreatic cancer and the typical prognosis with pancreatic cancer comes with a five-year, 5 percent survival rate."

So, believing that the likelihood of survival is slim, I run off to Thailand to spend my time and remaining resources in keeping with the five-year estimate of my demise. As my money runs out and I appear to be in good health, I return to my oncologist, who runs tests that reveal my titer of mutated pancreatic cells is now below the standard level classified as cancerous. Given our very litigious society, to my oncologist's dismay, I may soon be able to replenish my dwindling resources and then some by winning a lawsuit that as a result of the (mis)diagnosis, I thought I was soon to be dead and went off to spend my remaining days and my remaining money in the little time I supposedly had left. For these reasons, most doctors and insurance companies focus on providing and/or reimbursing for treatments of later-stage and harder-to-treat cancers rather than identifying and treating them in early stages.

We need to change this situation. The good news is that technology has helped produce a number of tests and devices that can help us. The bad news is that awareness of them is low and access is limited. Though I can certainly help raise awareness,

AI AND EARLY DETECTION

AI, or artificial intelligence, is a convenient (if perhaps not completely accurate) umbrella term to describe digital innovations pertaining to healthspan. AI is always learning and improving, and technologists are also continuously learning and improving their AI systems. Increasingly, AI will be used to continuously monitor all aspects of our bodies. It will allow us to measure the flux that is part of the human system; it will collect data that will tell us a particular food causes a harmful effect and another food a positive, beneficial one. It will tell us how exercise affects our sleep and our energy. By accumulating this type of data, we can adjust on the fly, giving us more control over our health.

it will take time, education, consumer demand, and technological advances before the promise of early detection and highly effective health monitoring is achieved.

I'm not going to cover every diagnostic innovation and digital medical application in this chapter, but I am going to focus on the ones that strike me as the most critical for health and longevity.

WHY MRI IS BETTER THAN PSA FOR DETECTING PROSTATE ISSUES

For years, doctors have used the prostate-specific antigen (PSA) blood test for prostate cancer screening. Even though it's still in widespread use, its effectiveness is questionable at best. It's telling that the inventor of the test, Richard Ablin, has admitted in a *New York Times* opinion piece titled "The Great Prostate Mistake"[37] that the test can show false positives and negatives and is therefore not reliable. Ablin wrote, "As I've been trying to make clear for many years now, PSA testing can't detect prostate cancer and, more importantly, it can't distinguish between the two types of prostate cancer: the one that will kill you and the one that won't." He and Ronald Piana eventually wrote the book *The Great Prostate Hoax*,[38] in which they chronicle the events and decisions that have led to its misuse.

Ablin's op-ed was published in 2010, but not much has changed since then. Part of the problem is that although a high PSA level may indicate prostate cancer and thus save lives, it comes with a heavy toll. If a prostate biopsy is then indicated, this procedure can cause incontinence and impotence. Is it worth it when approximately 15 percent of men with normal PSA tests have prostate cancer, and when a significant percentage with abnormal PSA levels don't? We know that PSA levels can be elevated by several factors unrelated to prostate cancer, from chronic prostatitis to bike riding before the test. Yet the American Urological Association still recommends PSA tests and insurance companies still pay for them, incentivizing their use. For legal reasons—meaning, quite frankly, to avoid the wrath and consequences of practicing counter to the "standard of care" and acknowledging that the emperor is not wearing clothes—even I've felt compelled to use PSA tests with patients.

The biggest problem I have with PSA tests is that a much better testing procedure exists: multiparametric MRIs. Most people are familiar with magnetic resonance imaging, which is a non–radiation-based, noninvasive test that uses a powerful magnet to align the body's protons with the magnetic field. By *multiparametric*, we mean that the device uses sequences from three different techniques to provide a more detailed view than a traditional MRI. The three imaging techniques—T2 weighted, diffusion weighted, and dynamic contrast enhancing—enable doctors to identify tissue types in the prostate, receive functional as well as anatomical data, and track the flow of blood using a contrasting agent which better reveals any cancer. All this communicates a tremendous amount of valuable information that allows doctors to gain more insight into what's happening with the prostate and to make better decisions.

While some people complain about the noise and feelings of claustrophobia in an MRI tube, it is a safe and accurate procedure. Though the patient must remain relatively still for twenty minutes or so, it is a "feet first" position and the head can remain outside the tube—unlike my aforementioned encounter being shoved head first into a children's MRI! A multiparametric MRI is far more accurate than either a PSA test or a digital rectal exam. The latter has little value, since it's such an imprecise, subjective test, and many doctors who administer it—by palpating the prostate through the anus with a gloved finger—lack the years of experience necessary to detect subtle, telltale signs of problems. It's akin to how it takes baseball hitters ten thousand swings before they become proficient; most doctors have not done anywhere close to ten thousand, or even *one thousand*, digital rectal exams.

Because of false positives, people often undergo invasive procedures like a biopsy that can cause unnecessary harm. A multiparametric MRI can detect lesions as small as five millimeters, which is quite tiny. Even better, software advances in Europe (particularly the Netherlands) enable technicians to spot lesions as small as three millimeters, an advance we can take advantage of by utilizing digital information transfer rather than having to travel to the Netherlands. As a result, this device can not only aid early detection but can guide the doctor's hand if a biopsy is necessary.

Multiparametric MRIs can help physicians assess whether watchful waiting is a viable option when a cancerous lesion is spotted, but is small. A significant percentage of prostate cancers are very small or grow slowly. In addition, quite a few prostate cancer patients are older or have comorbidities. These are all factors that may make watchful waiting a better alternative to surgery or other treatments. The MRI can allow us to observe suspicious lesions over time and determine if they're likely to metastasize.

Given all these benefits, why isn't this technology widely available?

The culprits are a lack of awareness and cost. The former is a problem not only for patients but for physicians; the information about multiparametric MRIs and prostate cancer communicated here isn't widely known even in the medical community. As a result, insurance companies generally don't cover the cost of this test, which can be considerable. My hope is that this situation will change as the medical community becomes more open to alternatives and aware of how they can save their patients' lives or at least prevent painful and unnecessary procedures.

BILATERAL CAROTID DOPPLER ULTRASOUND

A number of early detection tests are under development for not only cancer, but for heart disease and metabolic disease such as diabetes. For heart disease, carotid bilateral Doppler ultrasound is now starting to be used and is a tremendously effective new tool to detect arterial plaque. A "wand" is waved over the neck areas where the carotid arteries run, and the ultrasound technology detects the level of plaque buildup. Statistically (95 percent correlation), the amount of carotid artery plaque corresponds to the amount of coronary artery plaque. Thus, patients can receive an early warning and act before the plaque becomes dangerous.

THE BEST TEST FOR DETECTING CANCER EARLY: ONCOBLOT

I know I'm harping on this point, but for good reason: *early detection of cancer often turns it into a manageable, nonfatal disease.* The problem has been that we don't catch the cancer until it has spread and become much more difficult to control. This is how Death gets the upper hand. People inside and outside of the medical community tend to ignore the biggest risk factor for most diseases: age. Instead, we often focus heavily on more controllable, but often less impactful factors for cancer such as diet, exercise, rest, and lifestyle choices. While these controllable factors are important, many patients have been known to ignore early signs of cancer because they're "doing all the right things" and thus postpone earlier screening. Unless one has a first-degree relative with cancer or another disease, such as CAD, these early detection screenings are typically low yield until age fifty. Then it makes sense to begin screening so that these cancers and other pathologies can be caught and treated early and effectively.

But what if we had a simple blood test that could serve as an early warning system for cancer? In fact, such a test exists—or at least it did. Let me explain.

Dr. James Morré was a professor of biochemistry and molecular genetics at Purdue, and he, along with his wife, Dr. Dorothy Morré, began studying how an herbicide created uncontrolled growth in a plant. He assumed that if he could understand the process by which the plant grew abnormally, he might gain insights into how cancer grows and spreads.

As I noted earlier, ENOX2 is a protein that is found only in cancerous tissues and fetal cells. Dr. Morré identified this protein and spent almost forty years studying it, publishing a textbook on ENOX2 proteins. Based on this extensive knowledge, he was able to invent a test that identified twenty-five cancers using ENOX2 including: bladder, colon, esophageal, breast, kidney, lung, lymphoma, melanoma, ovarian, pancreatic, thyroid, testicular, and others. It was called the ONCOblot.

By using antibodies to the ENOX2 protein, the ONCOblot creates a plot on a western blot that identifies the weight and pH of the ENOX2 protein. This process allows the ONCOblot to figure out the cancer of origin, even for cancers as small as one millimeter, which is roughly the size of a needle's tip. In other words, it can find cancers in their early stages, even earlier than the multiparametric MRI which, even with the most advanced software, can only spot them at three millimeters.

I've used the ONCOblot with patients and it has been highly effective in identifying various cancers which were later confirmed by more traditional tests and procedures. In the instances when ONCOblot has detected an early cancer that hadn't been confirmed initially by traditional approaches, it was because traditional methods were unable to detect cancers as small as the ones identified by the ONCOblot; only when the cancers grew were the traditional methods able to confirm the ONCOblot findings.

Given the almost miraculous capability of the ONCOblot test, it's tragic that it's no longer available. After James Morré passed away, Dorothy sold the rights to the test to a partner in their investment group, a Chinese billionaire who, for whatever reasons—not the least of which is the exorbitant amount of time and money required to acquire FDA approval—has chosen not to make the test available in the US. Fortunately, another group has been working on replicating the ONCOblot process and indications are that their process will be a new and improved version. It is reported that their approach not only will identify all the same early cancers as the ONCOblot, but will also be capable of staging them. Though it's not on the market as of this writing, it soon will be, and the further good news is that it will not require a western blot. Therefore, the test will be approximately 20 percent or less of the cost, will be easily replicated, and will deliver results more quickly. This test can make a huge difference in how we treat cancer.

While the ONCOBlot is not readily available now, we do currently have GRAIL in the United States, a liquid biopsy (blood test) for the early detection of some cancers. However, it costs close to $1,000 per test and is not as sensitive as we would like. Nevertheless, it is a great start and gives us something to fill the gap left by ONCOblot. In addition, we have other tests such as RGCC and nagalase that help us identify and treat cancers early on.

Too often, we tend to think about cancer in terms of cures. As most people are aware, the growth and spread of cancer is like a runaway train—it's incredibly difficult to stop. But what if we had an indication that the train was about to accelerate and barrel down the track? We could divert it to an abandoned sidetrack where it would do no harm.

It's been estimated that if everyone had regular colonoscopies starting at the age of fifty, we could cure or prevent the vast majority of colon cancers. While it's premature to make the same statement about an ONCOblot-like test, it could potentially have an enormously positive effect on the treatment and prevention of a wide range of cancers if broadly adopted and studies confirm the results. From a healthspan perspective, it's tremendously positive news.

ARTIFICIAL INTELLIGENCE GETTING SMARTER

If you recall the original *Star Trek*, when someone would become ill or was injured, Dr. Leonard "Bones" McCoy would wave a diagnostic scanner over their bodies and immediately receive an accurate diagnosis. Then, Bones would often cure his patient with a single shot.

In the mid-sixties, when the show was made, such diagnosis and treatment might have been called futuristic. Today, the future is starting to arrive: AI is changing how we diagnose and treat patients and we're making incredible, swift advances in this area. AI's ability to hold and process huge amounts of information is especially useful today in helping doctors evaluate images. For instance, AI can take numerous images of a cell mutation present in early-stage liver cancer and then identify these types of cells in a new image (such as an MRI scan) better and faster than even the most experienced doctor or technician. While AI is currently used as a complementary or even a lead tool, it is not yet being used alone. This situation will inevitably change and, while it's likely that AI will not replace radiologists, it will certainly transform the nature of their work in the near future. We're currently using "narrow AI," focusing its use on a single task or goal. In the future, we'll transition to "general AI" where it's used much more broadly as a diagnostic and decision-making tool for a range of conditions and purposes.

Look at the benefits of AI another way. Imagine a highly experienced doctor, in practice for forty years, who has treated many patients successfully and learned enough to qualify as an expert. Now imagine being able to draw on the knowledge and skills of *five thousand* other doctors with the same amount of experience and expertise. Better yet, imagine a tool that can store all this knowledge in a database, process and evaluate it in terms of a given disease or patient condition, and extract the right information for treatment in mere seconds.

In another use for AI, we're getting a glimpse of the monitoring and diagnostic potential of "wearables." The tech isn't there yet and the devices aren't particularly precise; the adage "garbage in, garbage out" (GIGO) unfortunately still applies for many current consumer wearables. We haven't found ways to input all the necessary data and variables needed for a highly useful output. The problems are many, some as simple as a wearable not being worn sufficiently tightly to provide accurate tracking. Others are not precise enough to be accurate. Another problem is that one size (of human and human body parts) doesn't fit all. People vary considerably in the data they produce, depending on their weight, the size of certain organs, and the way their bodies work as well as other factors. For example, one athlete may have a larger heart and greater ejection fraction than another athlete and this can throw off the evaluation of data from wearable trackers. It can also be difficult to evaluate data without enough data to pull from. To create a useful context, the types of measurements are just as important as the number of measurements.

BRAIN-COMPUTER INTERFACES

This may seem like speculative fiction, but researchers have already developed systems that can coordinate patients' thoughts with actions—helping people who have lost an arm use an artificial one as if it were the one they were born with. Successful experiments have also been conducted in which computers can "read" the brains of people who have lost the ability to speak, translating what they're thinking into words. The potential to restore partial or complete function for people with disabilities is tremendously exciting and this technology may someday be applied to help survivors of debilitating spinal cord injuries. AI-powered bionics could lead to the creation of "smart" replacement body parts.

Another problem is that not all wearables collect "the right data." For instance, one monitor may measure body temperature and sleep stages better than others, but another may better measure movement and oxygen saturation, so people would need both devices for a full picture. We are left simultaneously using chest-strap heart-rate monitors to accurately measure heartbeats per minute, watches with accelerometers for accurate measurement of steps, rings for accurate measurement of data associated with stages of sleep—each with its own unique benefit but none with all of the best technology rolled into one. Bones's single, do-it-all medical wand is, for the moment, still beyond the medical final frontier.

Nonetheless, the wearables market is exploding, and that's yielding at least some healthspan benefits. Even if the measurables aren't always accurate, they raise users' consciousness about important health factors like heart rate, sleep quality and quantity, blood sugar (via continuous monitoring), and so on. Ideally, this increased consciousness will result in better diets, more effective and efficient exercise, and a stronger commitment to getting a good night's sleep. In terms of valuable health data, some wearables can collect fairly precise measurements of temperature, respiration, blood oxygen saturation, heart rate, blood pressure, and electricity-measured ECG readings (sinus rhythm and atrial fibrillation). Heeding this data can alert patients and doctors to problems while motivating healthier behaviors.

Invariably, AI and related technologies will advance far beyond the current state of wearables. Already, we're seeing companies progress beyond offering wrist bands and chest straps. You can also purchase devices such as stamps and skins or earplugs that can be worn on or in the body to deliver data about blood sugar, cortisol, electrolytes, lactate, uric acid, glycine, ammonium, and other key health measures.

THE BEST DEVICES FOR GAINING THE HEALTH ADVANTAGE

As of this writing, here are the digital devices that seem to be having the most benefits for healthspan:

- *Oura Ring.* Made by a Finnish company, this convenient ring tracks data that correlates at over 90 percent to the output of an EEG, the gold standard for sleep evaluation. It has become smaller over time—currently the size of a wedding band—and provides additional information about pulse rate, temperature, calories burned, and so on.
- *Apple Watch.* I prefer this watch to competitors' devices because it works well with other Apple products, though Fitbit and Garmin make equally good ones. They all track activity with an accelerometer (which helps determine the movement and intensity of your workout) and measure heart rate. These devices do a good job of monitoring vital signs continuously during workouts, though for more serious athletes, the chest and forearm straps provided by Polar H10 and Wahoo are better for more precisely tracking heart rate.
- *BioStamp from MC10.* This will soon be on the market and is for people who want to dig deep into their health. This device has a sensor that conforms and adheres to at least twenty-five body locations and offers metrics to evaluate sleep, posture, activity, and vital signs. The measurements are of medical quality and can be used for clinical evaluation. Currently, MC10 has limited distribution for clinical trial use, but given its uniqueness and marketability, it should have wider distribution in the near future. This limited availability also makes it expensive, though the cost presumably will drop as distribution expands.

With these devices come various mobile applications that directly tie to the devices or indirectly tie via an application programming interface to multiple devices. These apps allow one to easily track various metrics of exercise, sleep, activity (or lack thereof), and so forth through their matching devices or connectivity with other devices and/or apps. For example, heart rate variability is an interesting metric for those interested in evaluating their autonomic nervous state. If one's sympathetic nervous system is more engaged, there tends to be less variability in the very small fraction of time between heartbeats versus if one's parasympathetic system were engaged. Because spending most of our time in the parasympathetic mode is better for thriving from a healthspan perspective—recovering, regenerating, repairing—we can look to our heart rate variability (HRV) score to gauge whether what we are doing, or have been doing recently, is furthering one system over another and presumably furthering or diminishing our healthspan. While healthspan has not yet been linked directly to HRV through studies, except that those with chronically low HRV scores below 15 tend to have reduced healthspan, HRV nevertheless provides useful feedback as to our autonomic nervous system state. This evaluation can then be incorporated with one's exercise tracking app to help measure the effect on one's body of recent workouts and whether to adjust the current day's workout based on this feedback and one's goals.

Tracking "data" such as exercise metrics, including heart rate, exercise minutes and distance, power output, calories expended, and steps, as well as foods and beverages eaten and calories consumed, can provide a general measure of our progress and adherence to a nutrition and exercise regimen. Unfortunately, the issue of accuracy and precision of wearables is still present for exercise, as well as the issue of recall and recording measurements of food and beverage for nutrition. Still, the very act of being mindful is worthwhile and often both revealing and motivating. Lots of people don't realize how many (or few) steps they actually take each day or, by making the effort to record it, how many calories they are actually eating between meals with a handful of nuts here and a half a glass of juice there. It can be enlightening and empowering at once and usually very motivating.

Here is a partial list of available and useful healthspan apps that I use and recommend, beyond the apps that accompany the devices just mentioned.

EXERCISE

- *TrainingPeaks*: Originally developed for bicyclists and runners, this app can actually incorporate all manner of exercise, with capabilities to analyze data from the basic to the very detailed. Importantly, this app also integrates with most of the other top exercise and nutrition apps.

- ***WahooX***: Developed for bicyclists using indoor "smart" trainers that include many "bells and whistles," including virtual course travel and calculations of power-to-weight ratios that are readily visible.
- ***TrainerRoad***: Developed for bicyclists using indoor "smart" trainers; comes with predesigned workouts but also provides the capability to create one's own.

NUTRITION

- ***MyFitnessPal***: For tracking every morsel or drop of food and beverage that crosses one's lips. This app has an extensive library of prepared and packaged as well as unprepared foods and beverages and their caloric content. Note that while this and other apps track the calories as stated on package labels, the labels' measurements themselves can be inaccurate by as much as 30 percent.
- ***Apple Health and Fitness apps***: Provided with Apple's iPhone and Apple Watch, these are both robust and tie to most available health-related apps. To date, there is no "all-in-one" app that ties all data sources together, though I am working on remedying this as I write. Because Apple's Health or Fitness apps can work with so many apps, however, these plus an iPhone (and, to a more limited degree, the Apple Watch) can often provide an interconnection workaround.

Of course, this is just the start of AI's revolutionary impact on medicine. Right now, the technology exists to increase the speed, accuracy, and efficiency of diagnosis. The real key, though, will be AI's ability to process data and draw correlations that can be tested. This is already happening with the development of drugs. We can evaluate a particular virus or bacteria for multiple characteristics that can lead to a possible solution, either developing a new drug or repurposing an existing one with the potential to combat the virus or bacteria. Without AI, the process of observing and evaluating the multitude of pathogens as well as the various drugs and structures to make potential drugs can take decades to identify. AI can do it much more quickly with some evaluations that can take only *minutes*! In the current pandemic, scientists have used AI to examine the potential for human genetic variants that can slow or accelerate the course of COVID-19. Labs tested these models in vitro to validate AI predictions of which drugs would be helpful in slowing virus replication and the mechanism of action.

More significantly, AI has helped generate at least eight different types of COVID-19 vaccine. Without machine-learning systems and lightning-fast computational analyses provided by AI, developing the vaccine candidates—especially the nonconventional, experimental ones—probably would have taken many months if not years.

Don't get me wrong; AI is not the complete solution to this and other healthcare challenges. Perhaps the best cautionary tale is that of IBM's Watson computing system and oncology. Watson was tasked with digesting all the collected data relating to cancer in the hope that it could identify patterns that might be useful for treatment. Yet, after Watson finished reviewing all the studies and other literature, its recommendations were not particularly useful. Though it could absorb and process information faster and in greater volume than any human being, it lacked the discernment of an experienced oncologist who could find applicable nuggets amid all the information. AI also isn't a substitute for the necessary lab and clinical studies; it can't shorten the time needed to test vaccines on animals and then humans, but it does accelerate theoretical aspects of development, at times with blinding speed.

The possibilities may not be endless, but they are wide ranging. The University of San Francisco Parnassus Campus is using the Oura Ring with volunteers (including myself) to track data acquired by wearers during the pandemic, assessing whether some of the metrics indicate people were infected before becoming symptomatic and testing positive for the virus. In the past, we've struggled with this type of data collection. Now, with wearables becoming much more common, we can obtain more and better data with great speed and AI can help us make correlations that lead to better methods of prevention and treatment—not just for COVID, but also for many other diseases and disorders.

AI can be a game changer, applicable to preventive, anti-aging, and traditional medicine. It will help us connect the dots between theory and both observable and quantifiable data points, especially ones in the area of biological aging and associated biomarkers.

Improving Your Health Future
with Gene Editing

WHO *DOESN'T* WANT to improve the genetic hand they've been dealt?

Wouldn't that be the best way to cheat Death?

The genes we inherit may increase the odds that we'll suffer from a given disorder or disease; they may make us more likely to have heart problems at a young age, or breast cancer, diabetes, and so on. Until relatively recently, there hasn't been much we could do about the possibility of playing with a stacked deck.

With the advances made in gene therapy, however, we now possess a tool that can alter our genes to help us beat the odds of negative health outcomes. Though we still have a ways to go before we can change DNA to prevent any disease or fight a given disorder more effectively, we've made astonishing progress in this area. Hundreds of clinical trials are being conducted in the gene therapy area (see clinicaltrials.gov) and the FDA has approved a limited number of gene therapy products. In July 2020, for instance, the FDA approved Tecartus, a cell-based gene therapy to treat a type of lymphoma. While results with Tecartus and other gene therapies can be modest, these along with more successful drugs show the "proof of concept" and the potential for dynamic results in the future. A list of approved products for a variety of conditions can be found at www.genetherapynet.com.

GENOME MAPPING PROVIDES A LONGEVITY FUTURE

When we understand what specific genes do and how they're connected to each other, we possess incredibly valuable information that we can use to our benefit. For instance, during the COVID-19 pandemic, scientists discovered that the virus was less likely to affect people with specific gene types than those who lacked these genes. SARS-CoV-2 enters the cell body through ACE-2 receptor inhibitors, but people with the ACE I/D receptor-1 genetic mutation were less susceptible to developing COVID and suffering its effects. As we accumulate data about various genes and their connections, we'll be in a much better position to assess the risk of various diseases to patients and to design more effective treatments based on their genetic makeup.

Before we get into the specifics of various diseases that are currently treatable through gene editing, as well as ones with promising results in clinical trials, we need to define what gene editing is and how it works.

CRISPR CHANGE AGENTS

The most successful gene editing process as of this writing involves clustered regularly interspaced short palindromic repeats (CRISPR). CRISPR technology is a process; CRISPR itself refers to specific DNA strands that can be cut using the enzymatic protein CRISPR-associated protein 9 (Cas9). In lay terms, it's a technology that allows us to edit genomes by changing cellular DNA. For instance, if you have a genetically inherited disease or are genetically predisposed to develop a disease, CRISPR allows us to alter nucleotides by either simply deleting the gene that causes a disease or deleting and replacing it with edited DNA that will have beneficial effects. Different diseases require different approaches; sometimes deleting is all that is required, other times a different editing/replacement technique is necessary because deleting may create problems with other cells along with the cure.

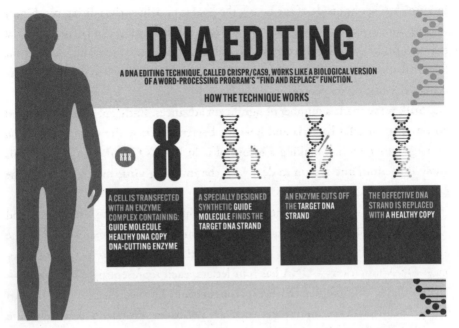

Overview of Gene (DNA) Editing Using CRISPR/CAS9 Technology

The size of the gene-editing tool affects its editing capabilities. This means that the "delivery vehicle" has to be large enough to accommodate all the editing tasks that are necessary. The usual delivery vehicle is an inactivated virus that contains the gene-editing material. If a gene requires three different deletions and insertions, it may be impossible for a single virus to contain all this material. Therefore, a series of treatments, rather than a single one, may be required or it may be advisable to find smaller editing tools to fit in the virus. Other options exist, but I want to convey that one size doesn't fit all—gene editing can be a varied process, depending on the disease being treated.

The potential of gene editing is staggering. Conceivably, it could be effective in helping people avoid everything from cancer to blood disorders to cystic fibrosis. Let me share a brief history of gene editing so you can see how much progress has been made in a relatively short period.

Scientists began testing various editing techniques in the 1970s, manipulating RNA and exploring the frontier of genome editing. Programmable nuclei were the early editing tools of choice until CRISPR was discovered and proved to be a superior technique, far easier to use and much more efficient. Whether done in vivo or in vitro (inside or outside of the body), the goal is to deliver the editing machinery to delete or correct targeted genes. Gene-editing studies ramped up considerably at the start of the twenty-first century. Out of an abundance of caution, much of the CRISPR testing focused on animals and bacteria, to ensure we do no harm before using gene editing on people.

Still, we've made a number of significant advances. Early on, scientists studied how a virus invades bacteria and how the bacteria destroy the virus but hold on to its genetic material, making a record of it in DNA's CRISPR sequences. This allowed the immune system to deal with the invading virus more effectively the next time it invades the bacteria.

This process provides scientists with insights about how to use viruses and CRISPR technology to reprogram DNA within cells. Over time, we've become much more sophisticated about these uses. Initially, we could only target single-letter DNA mutations—DNA has four letters, each representing a nucleotide—such as sickle cell anemia. With experimentation, however, we learned how to address multiple-letter mutations such as Tay-Sachs disease, a relatively rare inherited childhood disorder caused by genetic mutations that results in serious nerve damage.

GENE EDITING

The ability to alter the genome in order to prevent genetically inherited diseases or to use it as part of an anti-aging treatment is being studied and tested. Scientists in China recently published a paper in which they used CRISPR and extracted KAT7 from genetic material, which, when inactivated, reversed the premature aging of cells. As part of these studies, we're going to gain a great deal of epigenetic information—how genes are affected by what we do, from the foods we consume to the drugs we take to the exercises we incorporate into our routines. As we become smarter about this area, we will be in a better position to manipulate epigenetics for healthspan purposes.

POSSIBLE IMPACT OF GENE THERAPY IN THE BODY

While CRISPR is the main technology for gene editing today, we'll probably see a number of new technologies gain traction in the next few years, broadening the uses of gene therapy. However, as of this writing, these are the main diseases and areas targeted by gene editing in clinical trials or available for medical use.

CANCER

The process used here is called CAR-T cell therapy, or simply CAR-T. *CAR* stands for "chimeric antigen receptor," a specific type of signaling site on a cell's surface. A gene for this receptor is introduced to a patient's blood in the lab. The gene inserts itself into the patient's T cells (which are part of the immune system), causing the T cells to bind to and attack cancer cells when returned to the patient. Blood cancers are currently the major target of this type of therapy.

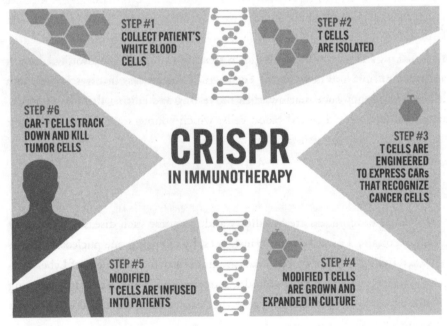

The Process of CAR-T Cell Therapy Using CRISPR

CAR-T therapy has been used quite a bit in the US and, though it's expensive, it's been effective. Tecartus, which I mentioned earlier, is a CAR-T therapy for lymphoma. About a half dozen CAR-T therapies have been FDA approved, though they haven't been found to significantly outperform traditional chemotherapy. While they do increase survivorship modestly in about 30 percent of cases, it comes with significant risks of cytokine release syndrome and destruction of B-cell function, which can lead to infection and sepsis.

The CAR-T process manipulates the patient's cells in the lab, but ideally we'll find a way to use allogeneic stem cells—cells from other people. We'll harvest stem cells from good candidates and alter them in the lab to fight cancer. The obstacle is preventing immune reactions to other people's cells, but I am optimistic we'll find a way around this sooner rather than later.

China has pioneered a different approach to cancer treatment using gene editing. Researchers there have used CRISPR to strengthen the reaction of T cells by removing the PD1 protein, which tumors can use to stop T cells from attacking. When CRISPR removes it, T cells are freed to attack and destroy the cancer.

BLOOD DISORDERS

Gene editing has also been successful in treating various blood disorders such as sickle cell anemia and hemophilia. For anemia, the process involves taking stem cells from patients' bone marrow, then harvesting and editing them so they produce fetal hemoglobin in red blood cells, which counters the disease's negative effect on these cells' oxygen-carrying capacity.

BLINDNESS

Many causes of blindness are hereditary and, for some such diseases, the culprit is a single mutated gene. In certain instances, by changing one nucleotide in the cell, the blindness can be cured. Trials are underway for treatment of Leber congenital amaurosis, which causes blindness during childhood. Scientists are using CRISPR to attack mutations in a gene that causes the disease and early results are promising.

HIV/AIDS

CRISPR technology has been used to treat HIV in clinical trials. In fact, in China, they have done gene editing in embryos, inserting a gene mutation called CCR5 that makes cells resistant to HIV.

MUSCULAR DYSTROPHY

At least two companies are working on this disease using gene editing. In the past, gene therapy struggled to address the causes of muscular dystrophy because back then you could only target one gene, an ineffective approach because muscular dystrophy is caused by multiple gene mutations. Now with CRISPR, we can target a number of them simultaneously, opening the door for possible treatments.

CYSTIC FIBROSIS

With this disease, mutations in the CFTR gene can produce severe respiratory problems. Gene therapy introduces a healthy version of the CFTR gene into patients, resulting in improved patient outcomes. While various approaches are still being tested, gene editing seems well suited for dealing with this type of genetic mutation.

HUNTINGTON'S DISEASE

Huntington's is a degenerative nerve disease—as nerves break down, everything from thought to movement becomes impaired. Typically, gene editing inserts a healthy gene into a cell in order to correct defects or supply what is missing. However, for this disease, gene therapy is designed to limit production of the Huntington protein that is causing nerve and brain damage. An enzyme is also introduced that guards against nerve damage, avoiding the "collateral damage" that can result from gene therapy for Huntington's.

* * *

This list is incomplete, of course. Many more diseases and disorders may benefit from gene editing in the future. Today, however, scientists are finding other applications for gene-editing technologies beyond treating or preventing specific diseases. Genetically modified organisms (GMOs) are a subject of controversy, but there are clear benefits—some foods are modified to allow people with allergic reactions (peanuts, eggs, etc.) to eat them. Gene editing is also being used to help animals, fruits, and vegetables become more resistant to diseases. Furthermore, scientists are using gene editing on pests (such as mosquitoes) so they can't breed or carry infectious diseases, which could reduce the heavy toll of malaria in developing countries.

To illustrate the breadth and scope of CRISPR technology, in what seems like the stuff of science fiction, there's even a group of scientists using gene editing in an attempt to bring the extinct wooly mammoth back to life. Their theory is that if they can edit the embryos of existing species that are genetically similar to mammoths, such as elephants, and combine them with genes from recovered wooly mammoth DNA, they may be able to edit genetically until they get the right match. This technique also may have applications in helping endangered species thrive.

CAUTIONS AND CONCERNS

Ultimately, gene editing is still in a developmental phase. Just as CRISPR represented a quantum leap in the technology, future leaps are likely to resolve some of the technique's current challenges, which I describe here.

First, the gene-editing process can result in genes crossing over into other cells. In fact, with CAR-T therapy, people have died in the testing phase because of this problem. Though CAR-T holds great promise for cancer patients, we're still trying to resolve the issue of healthy cells being attacked during immunotherapy treatment.

Second, ways to increase the size of the virus—or methods used to fit the gene-editing material in the virus—are still being debated and tested. Lambda Red is a recombination-mediated genetic engineering technique that is currently being researched and Integrase is another promising approach that helps insert viral DNA into chromosomal DNA. Nanotechnology also has potential for delivering more gene-editing material to cells. Nanoparticles of fat can carry gene editing through the bloodstream and, since most of the fat ends up in the liver, it can be used to target liver disease.

Third, we're still perfecting our gene-editing techniques. Prime Editing is an experimental technique that has generated a lot of early enthusiasm because it permits more precise genetic editing by conferring greater flexibility and control. This addresses another potential problem in genetic editing: damage to DNA strands when they're cut. Genetic editing can be done in different ways with varying pluses and minuses. Prime Editing, however, uses a specific, modified protein to replace a letter on a DNA strand without damaging it. Prime Editing or some other version of it may replace CRISPR as the gold standard.

Fourth, and perhaps most troublingly, people in certain religious communities have spoken out against genetic editing. Their argument is that genetic editing interferes with God's plan; that when we start changing a person's genetic makeup, we've crossed a line. When I heard this argument, I responded by telling a story about the man in the flood. As the waters began to rise, the man refused law enforcement directives to leave the area, stating that "God will save me." As the water level rose to the point where he could no longer leave by land, the man refused help from rescuers in a boat, repeating, "God will save me." As he stood on the top of his roof because the water had engulfed most of his house, the man refused a rescue by helicopter and again said, "God will save me." When the man ultimately faced God in Heaven, he asked why God had not saved him, and God replied, "What more do you want from me? I sent you a law enforcement officer to get you to leave, and a boat and a helicopter to rescue you!"

Whether God or science has given us the technology, my belief is that its existence justifies using it to save lives. Yes, we need to be ethical about our practices and we need to inform people in clinical trials about the risks in the genetic-editing process. We also must acknowledge that it's too early to know what the long-term effects of these genetic therapies might be. But think about it this way: Alzheimer's is a terrible disease and if you have the gene APOE-e4, your odds of getting this disease increase dramatically. Scientists are currently doing research in which they've used CRISPR to alter the gene in nerve cells that decreases production of a protein associated with Alzheimer's. Though there's no guarantee this will result in a cure, if it would safely reduce your odds of getting the disease, wouldn't you be willing to overcome your philosophical or religious objections and have doctors do the gene editing?

KNOW YOUR GENOME

I would be remiss if I didn't mention a product related to genetic editing that is also an affordable and worthwhile healthspan tool.

In recent years, we've seen a number of companies offering genetic testing directly to the public. Companies like 23andMe have successfully marketed themselves by promising to analyze DNA and tell people everything from the diseases to which they're susceptible to their ancestry. A company like Promethease is especially adept at filtering the data so that it can be used diagnostically. While some genetic testing companies may be more reputable than others, mapping one's genome is a good healthspan decision.

One of the benefits is knowing how people might respond to certain medications. Genome testing can identify an individual's SNPs—single-nucleotide polymorphisms, or DNA variations within a nucleotide. Scientists have been busy identifying them because certain ones can predict people's susceptibility to diseases and how they react to specific drugs. For instance, we know that one SNP diminishes the effectiveness of losartan, the blood pressure medication. We know that individuals with an ACE1 I/D mutation are less susceptible to COVID than others (though it also makes them less responsive to ACE-receptor blood pressure medication). We also have done sufficient testing to be aware of which diabetes medications are more or less effective, depending on one's genome. When people possess the rare DEC2 SNP, they can sleep fewer hours than recommended without suffering any ill effects. Genomind is a "precision medicine" company that focuses on matching the best medication to the individual's diagnosis using that individual's genome to identify related SNPs.

In the future, we won't have a one-size-fits-all approach to prescribing drugs. We'll recognize, for example, that for a given condition, the preferred medication is only effective for 80 percent of the population with a specific DNA makeup, and that the other 20 percent should receive an alternative drug.

The entire field of genetics is evolving rapidly, and though it's impossible to predict exactly which diseases can best be targeted, we can predict that advances like CRISPR will help many of us live longer and better.

Living Even Longer and Better in the Future

THE FIELD OF regenerative/anti-aging medicine is exploding, attracting the interest of big businesses that are investing major dollars. Apple is pouring money into a variety of health and wellness services, including health-monitoring wearables such as its Apple Watch. Amazon is making forays into the pharmaceuticals business. Google's website features a bold commitment to "transform the future of health."

Smaller but well-funded entrepreneurial businesses are also investing in a wide range of areas, including AI, supplements, and nanotechnology. Invariably, they will improve on many of the pioneering efforts of those who came before them.

Here is just a sampling of developments on the horizon:

- AgeX is on the verge of developing technology to reverse the age of a human cell and regenerate injured tissue through its trademarked stem cell technology called iTR (induced tissue regeneration).
- Geron is using its knowledge of telomeres to kill cancer cells and treat other diseases such as HIV, as well as reverse and slow cellular senescence.

- Various drug manufacturers are using AI to develop senolytic drugs (described hereafter) targeting age-related diseases and mTOR inhibitors that have potential in the fight against cancer.

As optimistic as I am about the results of all this money and expertise being focused on healthspan-related research, I also recognize that these efforts can be problematic. While most of the projects are well intended, some seem off the mark; companies are investigating products that are tangential to regenerative medicine or are affected by researcher bias. In addition, there's bound to be some missteps along the way, in the form of promising, well-publicized studies that raise expectations only to dash them when projects don't pan out. The coronavirus pandemic provides a microcosm of these thwarted expectations. Initially, therapies such as hydroxychloroquine or convalescent plasma were thought to be potentially breakthrough treatments, but they turned out to be ineffective. We need to recognize that not all promising treatments will fulfill their promise.

And of course, regulatory approval for various products and procedures will continue to be an obstacle.

Nonetheless, healthspan is a concept that has entered the public consciousness, as evidenced by the change in how we perceive aging. For years, aging was treated as an inevitable decline toward demise with no possible treatment. Today, it's viewed by many as a disease, and research is focusing on treatment. Though some speculate that the maximum lifespan in an ideal future is 150 years, this age maximum will likely increase even more as we make quantum leaps in gene editing, stem cell treatments, and other areas.

Let's look at some specific spheres where we're likely to see more innovative, effective, and potentially breakthrough developments.

PRE-DIFFERENTIATING, REPROGRAMMING, RECONDITIONING

We don't always have to invent a better mousetrap. We possess many effective drugs and other treatments, but the ways we administer them are not always optimal. A great deal of work is being devoted to improving delivery methods. Nanotechnology has received considerable attention recently because of its use in delivering coronavirus vaccines, and it holds immense promise for other types of treatments.

Regenerative researchers are investigating other "tweaks" that increase the efficacy of existing treatments. Though injecting stem cells has become standard regenerative therapy, we're always looking to improve stem cell effectiveness and one way of doing so is by pre-differentiating these cells. If you're using stem cells to strengthen the heart muscle, you would remove heart tissue from the patient, put it in a petri dish for a few days so that it differentiates into a cardiac myocyte (heart muscle cells), and then reintroduce it into the body—it will go straight to the heart muscle. This may be an especially useful technique for neurological issues, where the blood–brain barrier poses an obstacle for stem cell treatment. Pre-differentiation may help overcome this obstacle and avoid the side effect (in about 25 percent of the cases) of tumor development. Similarly, researchers are pre-differentiating stem cells into cartilage tissue to prevent development of bone-on-bone arthritis, hoping to prevent surgical procedures that require long recovery and incur major costs.

Reconditioning and reprogramming are two other promising areas of research. Molecular biologists experiment with cells, repairing them so they perform almost as good as new, or redirecting them to provide specific health benefits. These processes can involve fixing cell mitochondria, activating nitric oxides, and other approaches. In experiments with mice, Stanford University researchers have taken the blood from young mice and infused it into older mice, rejuvenating the older mice—the blood protein albumin seems to play a key role in the anti-aging effect.

As exciting as this future is, you should also be aware of what can slow down or even stop these developments from becoming effective regenerative medicine treatments.

• • •

STAYING AHEAD OF THE INFORMATION

For those who are interested, a website exists (clinicaltrials.gov) that provides information about different studies for a wide range of conditions and diseases. You can type in the term in which you're interested, and you'll be directed to relevant studies. While the treatments won't be available immediately (and may never be available—a lot of testing and regulatory hurdles stand in the way), you can see what could be available in the future.

POTENTIAL OBSTACLES AND HOW TO OVERCOME THEM

Breakthroughs don't happen overnight. Scientific research is, by definition, a slow process, demanding rigorous analysis and checking and rechecking results. Time, therefore, is a kind of obstacle, one that frustrates all of us who see exciting results in the lab and are eager to translate them into treatments for our patients. But as physicians, "Do no harm" is our mantra, and so we are extremely slow and careful before we're willing to use an experimental approach (no matter how spectacular the research might be) on human beings.

Besides time, here are some other obstacles that stand in the way of turning promising research into practice:

- *Traditional medical methodology.* In 1993, science journalist Gary Taubes published a book titled *Bad Science*, in which he documents the "discovery" of cold fusion. In the book, Taubes highlights the many mistakes that were made in the research and how the researchers' biases crept into their experiments and produced false conclusions. In the same way, some medical researchers also practice bad science—they are biased (whether consciously or not), aren't sufficiently precise in their experiments, fail to invest sufficient time or money in testing, and so on. Again, think about how many mistakes were made when it came to finding treatments for COVID. Just because we want a given drug to be a cure doesn't mean it will be one. We need to develop better research methodology, screening out biases, attracting funding for the most promising tests, and identifying the advantages and disadvantages of a given treatment with objectivity and thoroughness.

- *Insurance companies/regulatory approval.* As I've noted in these pages, a number of effective diagnostic and treatment innovations are either not available or are prohibitively expensive, thus limiting availability. Part of the problem is the reluctance of insurance companies to reimburse patients for treatment they deem "experimental"; another issue is the snail-slow regulatory-approval process. Perhaps the relatively rapid approval of COVID vaccines demonstrates that moving quickly and testing for safety aren't necessarily mutually exclusive. And while this particular approval was emergent in the face of a global pandemic in order to arrest accelerating death rates (with formal approval following months later), there's reason to hope that a medium approach could be obtained—somewhere between the rapid emergency approval of COVID vaccines and the more plodding approach the FDA seems to take for almost all other drugs, especially when it can be proved that death resulting from a particular drug's use is not imminent.

- ***Ballyhooed treatments and products that turn out to be ineffective.*** Nothing hurts advances in a given health sector more than rising expectations for a product being met by harsh realities that dash these expectations. In June 2021, Biogen received FDA approval for an Alzheimer's drug. Unfortunately, this drug's effectiveness has been questioned by a number of experts, and the FDA mandated that Biogen perform a confirmatory trial (after three FDA panel members resigned over their initial approval of the drug) to establish the drug's relevance to treating Alzheimer's. Still, it may have received approval because so many people are desperate for something that works against Alzheimer's and some studies suggested the drug might provide a small benefit. The problem here is "the boy who cried wolf." If you tell people that Biogen's drug and others will help them and it doesn't, the skepticism will dampen enthusiasm for research that might actually produce something that works far more effectively. Also, as an important aside, a recent study shows that a fairly inexpensive generic drug, valacyclovir, can be used to help prevent, slow, and even reverse development of Alzheimer's disease. Yet I'll bet even most physicians are unaware of this, because there is no financially compelling reason for manufacturers of this drug to communicate this news.[39]

While I don't have solutions to all of these problems, I do believe that the rapidly growing interest in regenerative medicine will create a groundswell of support for products and treatments that impact healthspan. Baby boomers and even younger generations are increasingly focused on taking care of their bodies and being proactive about their health. Many of them embrace alternative therapies and want to live not only longer, but better. They will demand insurance coverage for new and emerging therapies, support political candidates who favor increased spending on health-related research, and protest when regulatory bodies drag their feet when it comes to promising drugs.

As a doctor, I'm sometimes frustrated that we don't make faster progress on clearing the obstacles we face. At American CryoStem, we applied for an

Investigative New Drug approval to use stem cells for treating concussion and pain; we cited many studies from other countries that offered ample evidence that this approach was effective, but still had to wade through a seemingly endless tangle of red tape. Part of the problem is that we lack coordination and integration of research groups worldwide that are working in the same or complementary areas. If we developed improved methods for sharing information and resources, we might be able to move forward faster. It would also help if we could reach universal agreement that aging is a treatable disease. We could then establish a specialty and overarching repository of information and authority to gather and integrate all the various research, speeding the process of discovery and treatment.

We also need more synergies between Big Pharma and smaller, more entrepreneurial research groups. Big Pharma can provide investment capital for research and development, but smaller companies often possess the knowledge, intellectual property, and talent to come up with innovative approaches in niche areas. Combining the two groups would benefit both and, more to the point, benefit society. If they were to join forces, research wouldn't only be driven by a financial desire to hit the home-run drug, but also by a more narrowly focused investigation into profitable treatments targeting the regenerative medicine market.

Furthermore, physicians need to do a better job of keeping current and not allowing insurance limitations to circumvent their medical judgment. These are complex issues and I don't pretend to have a solution, but I know that if doctors make a greater effort to inform themselves of new and emerging treatments and procedures, they can help usher in a golden age of regenerative medicine. Too many doctors are content to treat patients with only the knowledge gained in medical school and residencies, not bothering to educate themselves about all the changes that have occurred since those years. Many times, I've heard of doctors telling their patients that stem cells don't work or haven't been studied enough to be used effectively. In most instances, these doctors are discounting this therapy because they're unfamiliar with it. Rather than putting in the work to research it, they decide it's worthless because it wasn't part of their education when they were young physicians.

We need doctors to lose their God-like attitudes and adopt a much more patient-centric open-mindedness and inquisitiveness. This is especially important as we enter an age of medical discovery and potential breakthrough treatments. Doctors need to communicate honestly and frequently with both patients and other doctors about what they've learned, adding to the larger healthcare database and helping people explore their treatment options. And when they don't know the answer? They should be honest with patients and admit they don't know, rather than maintain a detrimental, all-knowing façade.

I recall early in my medical school training when I would shadow experienced doctors who would recommend third or fourth-best options to patients. When I asked these physicians why they were recommending less-than-optimal treatments, they would explain that the optimal treatments weren't covered by health insurance, while the ones recommended were. Variations on this theme still exist today. In some cases, insurance won't cover drugs, procedures, and other treatments that are the best options for patients. In other instances, the costs of comprehensive coverage are exorbitant, shutting out the patients who can't afford it. Again, I have no magical solution to all of the thorny health insurance issues. However, I do believe that doctors need to do a better job of controlling what we can control, which means being as up to date as possible about the range of products and procedures that are showing positive results, whether in clinical studies or in other countries.

Knowledge can be power. This book is my small way of contributing to the knowledge in the field of regenerative medicine. We are making great strides toward living longer, healing faster, and looking better. It is everyone's responsibility—patients, doctors, and other healthcare providers—to educate themselves about all the emerging, game-changing approaches. The more we know, the easier it will be for us to put our healthspan plans into practice.

Can we cheat Death? Yes, and not just by living longer. We can live with greater energy, with less pain, and with the ability to heal more quickly from injuries. We will gain power over our healthspans and our aging, living not only longer, but better.

ACKNOWLEDGMENTS

IF NOT FOR Bruce Wexler taking my usually scattered and punctuated nerd-speak and, with inquisitive notes and self-study, translating it into more articulate and understandable language, the content of this book would not have made it to print.

Without the team at BenBella providing their expertise to add a whole new level of polish and shine, the material and concepts in this book would not be received nearly as well if at all.

I must also thank Charlie Fusco and her team at TGC for all their help with simply getting what I would like to share with others "out there" in a way that is successful and adheres to my values. The TGC Team was also essential in organizing the content in a much more readable, relevant, and understandable way that is crucial in any writing, but particularly with scientific material such as this.

Then there is my team at RSM that helps me do what I love best—practice medicine—helping patients optimize their health and improve their healthspan. They understand that their role is equally as important as mine and that without them, none of us could help people as we do.

And to my patients and peers with a kindred spirit in and passion for improving healthspan and learning about and ferreting out all the ways to do so.

Finally, I must acknowledge three of my other family: my mother, who is the sweetest person I know, and my father, who is the best critical thinker I know. In life, we often don't know the value of things when we should, but looking back on my life, I realize I am lucky and blessed to have two loving parents who sacrificed much to prioritize being parents to me and my sisters. And to my wife, Melanie, who I am blessed to have as a friend, wife, and loyal companion, and as a counterbalance of stability to my hypomanic, too often thinly spread, and hyperintense self.

NOTES

1. For the first part of this series, and links to the other parts, visit https://peterattiamd .com/ns001/.
2. John P. A. Ionannidis, "Why Most Published Research Findings Are False," *PLoS Medicine* 2, no. 8 (2005): e124, https://doi.org/10.1371/journal.pmed.0020124.
3. Carlos Lópes-Otín, Maria A. Blasco, Linda Partridge, et al., "The Hallmarks of Aging," *Cell* 153, no. 6 (2013): 1194–1217, https://www.ncbi.nlm.nih.gov/pmc/articles /PMC3836174/.
4. David Lyons, "My Third Stem Cell Treatment for Multiple Sclerosis," DVCStem, November 23, 2021, https://www.dvcstem.com/post/dave-lyons-stem-cells.
5. Iacopo Chiodini, Davide Gatti, Davide Soranna et al., "Vitamin D Status and SARS-CoV-2 Infection and COVID-19 Clinical Outcomes," *Frontiers in Public Health* 22 (2021), https://www.frontiersin.org/articles/10.3389/fpubh.2021.736665/full.
6. "Dr. Kami Hoss, Leading Dental Expert, Highlights Impact of Oral Health on Overall Health Ahead of National Dental Care Month in May," *San Diego Downtown News,* April 25, 2022, https://sandiegodowntownnews.com/dr-kami -hoss-leading-dental-expert-highlights-impact-of-oral-health-on-overall-health -ahead-of-national-dental-care-month-in-may/.
7. National Cancer Institute, "Cancer Statistics," updated September 25, 2020, https:// www.cancer.gov/about-cancer/understanding/statistics.
8. Council for Responsible Nutrition, "2019 CRN Consumer Survey on Dietary Supplements," accessed July 22, 2022, https://www.crnusa.org/resources/2019 -crn-consumer-survey-dietary-supplements.
9. Keisuke Yaku, Keisuke Okabe, and Takashi Nakagawa, "NAD Metabolism: Implications in Aging and Longevity," *Aging Research Reviews* 47 (2018): 1–17.
10. Julie S. Jurenka, "Anti-inflammatory Properties of Curcumin, a Major Constituent of *Curcuma longa*: A Review of Preclinical and Clinical Research," *Alternative Medicine Review* 14, no. 2 (2009): 141–53.

11. Center for Biologics Evaluation and Research. "Approved Cellular and Gene Therapy Products." U.S. Food and Drug Administration, FDA, accessed August 2, 2022, https://www.fda.gov/vaccines-blood-biologics/cellular-gene-therapy-products/approved-cellular-and-gene-therapy-products.

12. Gary K. Steinberg, Douglas Kondziolka, Lawrence R. Wechsler, et al., "Clinical Outcomes of Transplanted Modified Bone Marrow–Derived Mesenchymal Stem Cells in Stroke: A Phase 1/2a Study," *Stroke* 47 (2016): 1817–24, https://www.ahajournals.org/doi/full/10.1161/STROKEAHA.116.012995.

13. Kurzweil, "Paralyzed Man Regains Use of Arms and Hands after Experimental Stem Cell Therapy," September 12, 2016, https://www.kurzweilai.net/paralyzed-man-regains-use-of-arms-and-hands-after-experimental-stem-cell-therapy; Amber Dance, "Stem Cell Therapy Gives Paralyzed Man Second Chance at Independence," USC Stem Cell, Keck School of Medicine of the University of Southern California, January 15, 2017, https://https://stemcell.keck.usc.edu/stem-cell-therapy-gives-paralyzed-man-second-chance-at-independence/.

14. California's Stem Cell Agency, "Stories of Hope," n.d., accessed February 17, 2021, https://www.cirm.ca.gov/patients/stories-hope.

15. Ying Liu, Dong-Lin Cao, Li-Bin Guo, et al., "Amniotic Stem Cell Transplantation Therapy for Type 1 Diabetes: A Case Report," *Journal of International Medical Research* 41, no. 4 (2013): 1370–77, https://journals.sagepub.com/doi/10.1177/0300060513487640.

16. Ashley Strickland, "After Experimental Treatment, 24-Year-Old Is Learning How to Live," *The Human Factor with Dr. Sanjay Gupta*, December 18, 2015, https://www.cnn.com/2015/12/18/health/turning-points-stem-cell-therapy/index.html.

17. Scott Brandt, "Patient from Denver Uses Stem Cells to Avoid Spinal Fusion & Heal Achilles, then Runs a Marathon," ThriveMD, June 19 2019, https://thrivemdclinic.com/patient-case-studies/avoid-back-surgery-heal-achilles/.

18. Amber Dance, "Stem Cell Therapy Gives Paralyzed Man Second Chance at Independence," USC Stem Cell, Keck School of Medicine of the University of Southern California, January 15, 2017, https://stemcell.keck.usc.edu/stem-cell-therapy-gives-paralyzed-man-second-chance-at-independence/.

19. International Society for Stem Cell Research, "About the ISSCR," accessed February 7, 2022, https://www.closerlookatstemcells.org/about-isscr/.

20. Alpha Stem Cell Clinic, "Clinical Trials," University of California, San Francisco, accessed February 7, 2022, https://stemcellclinic.ucsf.edu/clinical-trials.

21. Mayo Clinic Center for Regenerative Medicine, "Clinical Trials," accessed February 7, 2022, https://www.mayo.edu/research/centers-programs/center-regenerative-medicine/patient-care/clinical-trials.

22. Joanna Rymaszewska, Katarzyna M. Lion, Lilla Pawlik-Sobecka, et al., "Efficacy of the Whole-Body Cryotherapy as Add-on Therapy to Pharmacological Treatment of

Depression—A Randomized Controlled Trial," *Frontiers in Psychiatry*, June 9, 2020, https://www.frontiersin.org/articles/10.3389/fpsyt.2020.00522/full.

23. Adam S. Sprouse-Blum, Alexandria K. Gabriel, Jon P. Brown, et al., "Randomized Controlled Trial: Targeted Neck Cooling in the Treatment of the Migraine Patient," *Hawaii Journal of Medicine and Public Health* 72, no. 7 (2013): 237–41.

24. Jari A. Laukkanen, Tanjaniina Laukkanen, and Setor K. Kunutsor, "Cardiovascular and Other Health Benefits of Sauna Bathing: A Review of the Evidence," *Mayo Clinic Proceedings* 93, no. 8 (2018): 1111–21.

25. Isaac Peña-Villalobos, Ignacio Casanova-Maldonado, Pablo Lois, et al., "Hyperbaric Oxygen Increases Stem Cell Proliferation, Angiogenesis and Wound-Healing Ability of WJ-MSCs in Diabetic Mice," *Frontiers in Physiology* 9 (2018): 995.

26. C. A. Bannister, S. E. Holden, S. Jenkins-Jones, et al., "Can People with Type 2 Diabetes Live Longer Than Those Without? A Comparison of Mortality in People Initiated with Metformin or Sulphonylurea Monotherapy and Matched, Non-diabetic Controls," *Diabetes, Obesity and Metabolism* 16, no. 11 (2014): 1165–73.

27. Hong Yu, Xi Zhong, Peng Gao, et al., "The Potential Effect of Metformin on Cancer: An Umbrella Review," *Frontiers in Endocrinology* (2019), https://www.frontiersin.org/articles/10.3389/fendo.2019.00617/full.

28. Centers for Disease Control and Prevention, "New CDC Report: More than 100 Million Americans Have Diabetes or Prediabetes," July 18, 2017, https://www.cdc.gov/media/releases/2017/p0718-diabetes-report.html.

29. Chung Hsun-Huang, Wen-Chung Tsai, Miao-Sui Lin, et al., "The Promoting Effect of Pentadecapeptide BPC 157 on Tendon Healing Involves Tendon Outgrowth, Cell Survival, and Cell Migration," *Journal of Applied Physiology* (2011), https://journals.physiology.org/doi/full/10.1152/japplphysiol.00945.2010.

30. Sarah A. Deek, "BPC 157 as Potential Treatment for COVID-19," *Medical Hypotheses* 158 (2022): 110736, https://doi.org/10.1016/j.mehy.2021.110736.

31. Alexandra Flemming, "Immune-Boost for the Elderly," *Nature Reviews Immunology* 18 (2018): 543.

32. Daniel P. Andersson, Ylva Trolle Lagerros, Alessandra Grotta, Rino Bellocco, Mikael Lehtihet, and Martin J Holzmann, "Association between Treatment for Erectile Dysfunction and Death or Cardiovascular Outcomes after Myocardial Infarction," *Heart*, BMJ Publishing Group Ltd and British Cardiovascular Society, August 1, 2017, https://heart.bmj.com/content/103/16/1264.

33. Geoffrey Hackett, Peter W. Jones, Richard C. Strange, and Sudarshan Ramachandran, "Statin, Testosterone and Phosphodiesterase 5-Inhibitor Treatments and Age Related Mortality in Diabetes," *World Journal of Diabetes*, Baishideng Publishing Group Inc, March 15, 2017, https://www.ncbi.nlm.nih.gov/pmc/articles/PMC5348622/.

34. Rebecca Vigen, Colin I. O'Donnell, Anna E. Barón, et al., "Association of Testosterone Therapy with Mortality, Myocardial Infarction, and Stroke in Men with Low

Testosterone Levels," *JAMA* 310, no. 17 (2013): 1829–36, https://jamanetwork.com/journals/jama/fullarticle/1764051; William D. Finkle, Sander Greenland, Gregory K. Ridgeway, et al., "Increased Risk of Non-Fatal Myocardial Infarction Following Testosterone Therapy Prescription in Men," *PLOS One* (2014), https://doi.org/10.1371/journal.pone.0085805.

35. Abraham Morgentaler, "2016 Testosterone International Expert Consensus Recommendations: Mayo Clinic," accessed July 26, 2022, https://0008581.myregisteredwp.com/wp-content/uploads/sites/756/2017/02/2016-Testosterone-International-Expert-Consensus-Recommendations.pdf. https://pubmed.ncbi.nlm.nih.gov/26586191/. https://pubmed.ncbi.nlm.nih.gov/27313122/.

36. G. D. Sherman, J. S. Lerner, Robert A. Josephs, et al., "The Interaction of Testosterone and Cortisol Is Associated with Attained Status in Male Executives," *Journal of Personality and Social Psychology* 110, no. 6 (2016): 921–29, https://psycnet.apa.org/record/2015-38657-001.

37. Richard J. Ablin, "The Great Prostate Mistake," *New York Times,* March 9, 2010, https://www.nytimes.com/2010/03/10/opinion/10Ablin.html.

38. Richard J. Ablin and Ronald Piana, *The Great Prostate Hoax: How Big Medicine Hijacked the PSA Test and Caused a Public Health Disaster* (New York: St. Martin's Press, 2014).

39. M. A. Wozniak, A. P. Mee, and R. F. Itzhaki, "Herpes Simplex Virus Type 1 DNA Is Located Within Alzheimer's Disease Amyloid Plaques," *Journal of Pathology* 217, no. 1 (2009): 131–38, https://doi.org/10.1002/path.2449; William A. Eimer, Deepak Kumar Vijaya Kumar, Nanda Kumar Navalpur Shanmugam, et al., "Alzheimer's Disease-Associated β-Amyloid Is Rapidly Seeded by Herpesviridae to Protect against Brain Infection," *Neuron* 99, no. 1 (2018): 56–63, https://doi.org/10.1016/j.neuron.2018.06.030.

GLOSSARY

Ablation: A process by which tissue is removed from the body by scraping, peeling, or vaporizing a surface.

ACE I/D: Angiotensin-converting enzyme insertion/deletion polymorphism is a difference in a gene that regulates the production of enzymes which cleave or cut proteins. Increased expression of the ACE I/D gene can confer both immune and performance benefits.

Advanced Glycation End Products: Fats or proteins that retain sugar molecules, which results in oxidative or inflammatory processes that in turn can be markers for the onset of diabetes or arthritis.

Alzheimer's Disease: A common type of dementia or cognitive decline, associated with memory loss and a decreased ability to coherently respond to environmental stimuli.

Amphetamines: A class of mood-altering drugs that stimulate the mind and body. In some cases, they are selected for treating attention-deficit/hyperactivity disorder and obesity.

Anaerobic: A metabolic process that occurs in the absence of oxygen, as opposed to aerobic processes which occur in the presence of oxygen.

Andropause: From the Greek "andras," which means human male, and "pause," to cease or decline. Hence, typical age-related decline of testosterone in men can lead to fatigue, decreased performance, and less efficient metabolic and immune function, as well as the onset of various diseases.

Anemia: An absence of a sufficient number of red blood cells and hemoglobin, which decreases the ability for oxygen to be transported to tissues in the body.

Angiogram: A medical imaging technique that can use X-rays, computerized tomography, and magnetic resonance, along with contrast dyes, to take a high-resolution image of the heart, pursuant to detecting arterial blockages or deterioration.

Ankylosing Spondylitis: An inflammatory process that, over time, can cause bones in the spine to fuse together.

APOE ε4: This gene instructs the production of apolipoprotein ε, the prevalence of which is associated with an increased risk of neurocognitive decline.

Arrhythmia: An irregular heartbeat.

Artificial Intelligence: A computer software program that can perform some tasks typically done by humans.

Atmospheres: This measurement describes the pressure of air at sea level, at a temperature of 15 degrees Celsius.

Autoimmune: This term refers to a condition whereby one's immune system attacks one's own body, unprovoked by an externally obtained disease, overreacting to normal tissues within the body. Type 1 diabetes, multiple sclerosis, systemic lupus, and irritable bowel diseases are examples of the immune system attacking itself.

Autophagy: A process of removing or recycling damaged cellular components, which helps to ensure normal cellular function. Notably, an increase in blood ketones (beta-hydroxybutyrate) as a result of fasting or consuming a ketogenic diet, can be a sign of increased autophagy.

Benzodiazepines: A class of drugs that decrease nervous system signaling, leading to a tranquil state.

Berberine: Derived from the berberis shrub, and sometimes used in combination with or instead of metformin, this supplement has been demonstrated to lower blood sugar.

Bioidentical Hormone Replacement: The practice of assessing the entirety of a patient's endocrine system, and then optimizing their hormone balance either by stimulating increased hormone production or replacing a deficiency in hormone production to restore normal hormone levels.

Blood-Brain Barrier: A mesh of closely packed endothelial cells that only allow certain substances into the brain, such as oxygen, while barring entry of toxic compounds.

BMI (Body Mass Index): The ratio of one's height to one's weight, by way of dividing one's weight in kilograms by the square of one's height in meters, stratified by age. Generally speaking, a BMI of 18 to 25 is considered normal.

Body Composition: The distribution or percentage of lean muscle mass to fat mass of one's body. The measurement of body composition is a much more accurate assessment than that of body mass index and can be performed via MRI, DEXA Scan, calipers, or water displacement.

Calorie: A measurement that describes a unit of food energy. This unit of energy is described as the amount of heat required to raise a kilogram of water by one degree Celsius, when a bomb calorimeter device is used to burn one gram of a specific food item.

CBC (Complete Blood Count): A standard and commonly run blood assay (test) that measures one's red blood cells, white blood cells, and platelets (along with neutrophils, eosinophils, basophils, and monocytes), pursuant to receiving insight into any number of potential disease pathologies.

CBD (Cannabidiol): A key constituent of the marijuana plant that can downregulate systemic inflammation.

Cholesterol: A type of steroidal lipid (fat) found in foods, and in one's bloodstream, which is an essential component of cell membranes.

Choline: An essential nutrient for humans that plays a key role in the synthesis of phospholipids, which ensure cell membrane health.

Circadian Rhythm: Physiological responses to the wake–sleep cycle within a twenty-four-hour period, as part of the four biological rhythms (along with diurnal, ultradian, and infradian).

Cryotherapy: The use of acute doses of whole-body temperature reduction to stimulate recovery and regenerative processes in the body. This is achieved via exposing the entire body (up to one's neck) to cold temperatures in a chamber (usually in a standing position), typically for two to five minutes, at temperatures ranging from –100° to –140°C.

CFTR: Cystic fibrosis transmembrane conductance regulator is a protein responsible for regulating the flow of electrolytes (sodium) in and out of a cell membrane. A mutation in the gene that regulates this protein can cause cystic fibrosis, which inflicts severe damage to one's lungs.

Culture: An organic, nutrient-rich material, often made out of amino acids, glucose (sugar), vitamins, minerals, and sodium, on which cells can grow.

Cytosine: A nucleic acid found in DNA sequences, along with thymine, adenine, and guanine.

DASH (Dietary Approaches to Stop Hypertension) Diet: Composed of a nutritional protocol that emphasizes vegetables, fruits, and whole grains. Including fat-free or low-fat dairy products, fish, poultry, beans, and nuts, it limits foods that are high in saturated fat.

Daunorubicin: Used to treat leukemia, this growth inhibitor can have some seriously profound side effects on bone marrow.

DEC2 SNP: This basic helix-loop-helix domain containing single-nucleotide polymorphism regulates one's response to the sleep cycle, allowing one to sleep less and still feel rested. Very few humans have this genetic mutation.

Deforolimus: Also known as ridaforolimus, this growth inhibitor is used to treat patients with osteosarcoma (bone cancer.)

Doppler Ultrasound: High-resolution imaging that can create both still and moving pictures of the body's soft tissues by reflecting sound waves off the body's structures.

ENOX2: Ecto-NOX disulfide-thiol exchanger 2 is a protein expressed on a cell's surface membrane under conditions of cell growth and proliferation and is associated with disease pathologies such as cancer and endometriosis. ENOX2 can be detected in blood.

Epirubicin: Used to treat breast cancer patients, this drug is known to slow metastatic progression of breast cancer through the lymph nodes.

Ergogenic: Supplements or drugs that improve one's ability to recover and increase physical performance.

Everolimus: A cancer-inhibiting drug (trade name Afinitor) appropriate for hormone-positive breast cancer patients.

Fibroblast: A connective tissue cell capable of producing collagen.

Fibromyalgia: Persistent fatigue accompanied by intense musculoskeletal pain.

Follicle Stimulating Hormone: Released by the pituitary gland, and responsible for stimulating the production of sperm in men and ova (eggs) in women.

GABA: γ-Aminobutyric acid is a neurotransmitter that inhibits nervous system excitability.

Glutamate: Also called glutamic acid, glutamate is a key α-amino neurotransmitter and catalyst for protein synthesis.

Glycemic Index: A measure of how quickly a given carbohydrate can raise blood sugar, ranked on a scale of 1 to 100.

Glycemic Load: A measurement equivalent to 1 gram of glucose (carbohydrate) required to raise blood sugar, obtained by multiplying the food or beverage's glycemic index by the total number of carbohydrates in that food, then dividing by 100. Glycemic load is an excellent measure of the sustained impact a given food will have on metabolism.

Glycogen: Stored glucose (sugar) energy, which can reside in the liver and in muscle, then used when the body needs additional energy.

Glycolysis: The metabolic process by which glucose (carbohydrate, sugar) is broken down by enzymes.

Gynostemma: Also known as jiaogulan, this plant from Southeast Asia has been demonstrated to lower both blood sugar and cholesterol levels in humans.

Healthspan: In essence, healthspan represents the portion of a person's life wherein they are in optimal health. In this book, we explore how to extend this period of optimization for the entire duration of a person's life.

Hematocrit: A measure of the percentage of red blood cells in a volume of blood, composed of platelets, white blood cells, plasma, and red blood cells.

Hemoglobin: The protein in red blood cells that carries oxygen.

Hemophilia: A condition in which one's blood does not clot properly; even a small laceration can produce severe blood loss.

Histamine Receptor Blocker: A class of drugs that inhibit the production of stomach acid, preventing the formation of ulcers.

Hyaluronic Acid: A molecule that is one of the key elements of the body's connective tissue, it surrounds cells in a gelatinous matrix, stimulating the production of collagen and elastin, and ensuring that one's skin remains supple and moisturized.

Idarubicin: This antitumor antibiotic inhibits protein synthesis in tumor tissue. Typically used to treat leukemia patients.

IGF-1: Insulin-like growth factor 1 is a liver-produced hormone, not dissimilar in structure to insulin, which helps to regulate adolescent growth, and can also produce anabolic effects in adults.

Inositol: A sugar molecule that plays a crucial role in intracellular signaling in response to both hormones and neurotransmitters.

Insomnia: A condition described as the inability to sleep at all or for a normal duration.

KAT7: Histone acetyltransferase is an enzyme encoded by the KAT7 gene, which in turn is responsible for DNA replication pursuant to the formation of new blood cells from stem cells.

Krebs Cycle: Describes a series of chemical reactions that release energy from proteins, carbs, and fats (macronutrients).

L-Arginine: An amino acid responsible for building protein structures in the body, by way of stimulating the release of nitric oxide, insulin, and human growth hormone.

Libido: Described as one's sexual drive or desire. A loss of libido can be a marker of aging and disease.

L-Methionine: An amino acid that can be found in dairy and meat products. It plays an essential role in metabolic and immune functions.

Luteinizing Hormone: An enzyme produced by the anterior pituitary gland, responsible for stimulating the production of testosterone in men and ovulation in women.

Lyme Disease: A tick-borne inflammatory disease described by joint pain and fatigue. Left untreated, it can lead to neurological and cardiac disorders, though an appropriate course of antibiotics can resolve it.

Macrolide: A class of antibiotics that inhibits the formation of proteins in bacteria, thereby killing them. For example, erythromycin (a substitute drug for those allergic to penicillin) is a macrolide often prescribed to patients suffering from respiratory tract infections.

Macronutrient: A type of food, such as a protein, carbohydrate, or fat. Notably, 1 gram of protein contains 4 calories, 1 gram of carbohydrate contains 4 calories, and 1 gram of fat contains 9 calories.

McBurney's Point: This refers to the area on the lower right quadrant of one's abdomen at which tenderness is maximal in cases of acute appendicitis. Palpation (manual manipulation) of this area can act as a first-order assessment and diagnosis of acute appendicitis.

Messenger RNA: A single strand of ribonucleic acid that codes for specific amino acid sequences that regulate protein synthesis.

Metabolite: An end product of metabolism, either made or used by the body, that can break down chemical structures into smaller components.

Methionine: An amino acid that can be found in dairy and meat products. It plays an essential role in metabolic and immune functions.

Methyl Group: A basic unit of organic compounds, composed of three hydrogen atoms and a carbon atom, which can be added to or subtracted from protein complexes, regulating their function in a cell.

Methylation: When this biochemical process is occurring optimally, it regulates neurological, immune, metabolic, and cardiovascular processes. However, when methylation fails to occur optimally, it can degrade overall physiological function, yet another hallmark of aging.

Mitochondria: These membrane-bound organelles (specialized structures within a cell, such as a cell's nucleus) are the primary energy producers in a cell, which create the root units of energy in the body, adenosine triphosphate (ATP). Notably, a decline in mitochondrial function can foreshadow any number of disease processes, such as cancer and diabetes.

MRI (Magnetic Resonance Imaging): An imaging technique by which a patient lies prone on a gantry and is exposed to a magnetic field and radio waves, which produce a picture of their internal organs and tissues. MRI can be used to diagnose brain tumors and injury to internal organs.

mTOR Complexes 1 & 2: These distinct proteins of mTOR (mammalian or mechanistic targets of rapamycin) are responsible for nutrient energy sensing and IGF-1 activation, respectively.

mTOR: Mammalian target of rapamycin (the bacterium *Streptomyces hygroscopicus*) is a signaling pathway that activates gene transcription and protein synthesis. Notably, mTOR activates muscle growth, but when unregulated, plays a central role in the proliferation of cancer.

Multiple Sclerosis: A disabling autoimmune disease of the spinal cord and brain, whereby one begins to lose motor function and vision.

Muse Cell: Multilineage differentiating stress-enduring cells are often derived from umbilical cord tissue and are novel insofar that they are noncancerous and can turn into just about any cell type in the human body.

Mutation: An alteration in the structure of a gene's nucleic acid sequence, typically from a mistake in replication, or as a result of some external impact such as a carcinogen.

Myelomalacia: A relatively rare condition that results in a softening of the spinal cord. Often a patient may not be aware of this condition, though it is extremely serious and can even be deadly.

Nagalase: α-N-acetylgalactosaminidase is an enzyme secreted by cancer cells that can inhibit one's immune system from performing properly. Nagalase can be detected in blood.

Nanotechnology: The use of technology on an extremely small scale, such as molecular or atomic, for medical or industrial application. One example of nanotechnology is using various metals such as gold to deliver targeted cancer-fighting drugs.

NIH: The National Institutes of Health is the primary United States governmental body that performs biomedical public health research.

N-Methyl-D-Aspartate Receptor: These neuronal cell receptors receive L-glutamate as part of the brain's role in learning and memory.

NSAIDs: Nonsteroidal anti-inflammatory drugs are a class of pharmaceuticals (such as ibuprofen) that inhibit inflammatory processes systemically, in comparison to steroids such as cortisone and prednisone.

Orthoquinones: Also referred to as ortho-quinone methides, these compounds are derived from cinchona bark and can be used as cytotoxins to combat cancer.

Osteomyelitis: Infection of the bone.

Parkinson's Disease: A disorder of the nervous system, expressing itself via non-voluntary tremors and loss of balance, as a result of the degradation of the external covering (myelin sheath) of the nerves.

PD1: Programmed cell death protein 1 is expressed on the surface of immune cells, such as T and B cells. Cancer has the ability to inhibit PD1 expression, and hence "hide" from the immune system.

PED-5 Inhibitor: Phosphodiesterase type 5 inhibitors allow smooth muscle cells lining blood vessels to dilate, thereby increasing blood flow.

PPAR: Peroxisome proliferator-activated receptors regulate metabolism, as well as gene expression.

Prolactin: A protein-based hormone secreted by the pituitary gland, which stimulates milk production in women during pregnancy. High prolactin levels in men can lead to gynecomastia, an enlargement of tissue around the nipples.

Proteostasis: Protein homeostasis within a cell constitutes a barometer of overall cellular health. Degradation of the protein-building machinery within a cell, such as the misfolding of proteins, is a common hallmark of aging.

Proton Pump Inhibitor: A class of drugs that block the stomach's capacity to produce acid, preventing symptoms of heartburn.

Reactive Oxygen Species: An unstable oxygen-bearing molecule, which can damage the DNA of a cell; typically characterized as a free radical.

Regenerative Medicine: The practice of using medical interventions in the forms of sleep optimization, nutrition, exercise, supplementation, drugs, therapies, and procedures, for the purpose of regenerating human cells, tissues, and organs.

RGCC: Circulating tumor cells that break away from a primary tumor complex. These can be detected in blood and are used as a proxy for understanding the state of disease and the efficacy of a given cancer therapy.

Schizophrenia: A psychological condition described by disorganized behavior and speech, accompanied by delusion.

Secretagogue: A substance that induces or stimulates secretion; for example amino acids, which stimulate the production of human growth hormone.

Senescence: When a cell gradually begins to lose its ability to divide or grow. While senescent cells do not necessarily die immediately, they can accumulate in the body, often leading to the presentation of age-related indicators such as failing eyesight or loss of hearing.

Sermorelin: This peptide (amino acid) can be injected under the skin to upregulate the body's production of growth hormone.

Statin: A class of drugs that reduce triglycerides and cholesterol in the blood and liver.

Superoxide Dismutase: An enzyme crucial for antioxidant defense in the body.

Tecartus: Brexucabtagene autoleucel is a genetically modified, autologously derived immune T-cell that is introduced into leukemia patients to kill cancer cells.

Telomere: A protective region of DNA found at the ends of chromosomes that, over time, decreases in length and protective capacity. Telomeres can be used as a measure of one's biological age.

Temsirolimus: This antigrowth drug is used to treat patients with renal cell carcinoma (kidney cancer).

THC: Tetrahydrocannabinol is the primary active component of the marijuana plant, which can be used for managing pain.

Time of Flight: How long it takes for a subatomic particle to move from one sensor to another. This mathematical function is crucial for improving the sensitivity and resolution of PET/CT (positron emission tomography/computerized tomography) scans when imaging cancer in the human body.

Tocopherol: Vitamin E, which can be consumed as an antioxidant supplement.

Trendelenburg Position: An angle of inclination achieved on a surgical table or medical bed, often used in pelvic surgery and to treat shock, in which a patient lies on their back, face upward, with the pelvis higher than the head.

Triglyceride: A fatty acid that is a primary component in body fat, and can also be measured in blood, high amounts of which can indicate risk of heart disease.

Trypsin: A digestive enzyme found in the small intestine, which can also be synthesized from plants, bacteria, and fungus, and which aids in the digestion of protein.

Tufstin: This tetrapeptide (four-chain amino acid) is known to increase immune function and inhibit inflammatory processes.

VO$_2$ Max: A measure of the maximum rate of oxygen consumption while exercising, calculated in milliliters per kilogram per minute, stratified by age. Generally speaking, 42 is an average VO$_2$ max for men, and 33 for women.

INDEX

ABOUT THE AUTHOR

AFTER REPEATEDLY BEING told it was impossible, Dr. Rand McClain was accepted into medical school at the age of thirty-seven. Dr. McClain earned his medical degree at Western University and completed his internship at the University of Southern California's Keck School of Medicine Residency Program (USC California Hospital), and has worked with some of the best and original innovators in sports, rejuvenative, regenerative (anti-aging), cosmetic, and family medicine. As the founder of Regenerative and Sports Medicine (RSM), Dr. McClain works with elite athletes, celebrities, CEOs, and anyone else who wants to make the most of what is available to optimize their health. He is a Medical Advisor to Vytalyx (a.k.a. DeepHive), an AI-based medical company utilizing blockchain technology to provide health professionals with unfettered access to intelligence and data for clinical wellness, and is a member of the Medical Advisory Board for American CryoStem, leaders in stem cell technology. Dr. McClain serves as part of the Medical Advisory Board of Z.E.N. Foods, and as the Chief Medical Officer for LCR Health supplements, and serves on the Board of Medical Advisors for Maximus, a men's sexual health telemedicine company. Additionally, Dr. McClain is a media staple, with frequent appearances on TV, radio, podcasts, and online features around all things health and longevity. He lives in Malibu, California.